MEDICINE TODAY,

HEALING TOMORROW

MEDICINE TODAY, HEALING TOMORROW

Dolph Ornstein, M.D.

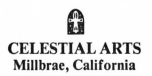

CELESTIAL ARTS
Millbrae, California

Grateful acknowledgment is made to Builders of the Adytum, 5105 No. Figueroa St., Los Angeles, California 90042, for permission to use their "Meditation on Aleph" from *The Book of Tokens* by Paul Foster Case.

Illustrations by Mary Elizabeth Bruno

CELESTIAL ARTS
231 Adrian Road
Millbrae, California 94030

First Printing, April 1977
Made in the United States of America

Library of Congress Cataloging in Publication Data

Ornstein, Dolph, 1947—
    Medicine today, healing tomorrow.

        1. Medicine—Philosophy.   2. Hygiene—Philosophy.
1. Title
R723.076   610'.1   76-53339
ISBN: 0-89087-173-6

1 2 3 4 5 6 7 8 — 82 81 80 79 78 77

Preface

It is said that we have just entered into the beginning of the Aquarian Age, an age of growth in love and beauty, versus the past two thousand years of the Picean Age characterized by self-sacrifice and guilt. It seems hardly apparent that the entire universe is in a process of change toward self-understanding, and spiritual unfoldment. In other words, towards a more meaningful life expression. Life is energy which substantiates everything.

Our body, which is a most miraculous creation, is a temple or vehicle in which we live and in which our thoughts manifest themselves. Our psyche governed by our conscious thoughts bring about the physical actions. It is therefore essential how we think and what we believe in. Life always is and cannot be destroyed, it can only change. To be healthy is thinking healthy and positive. We have the power to change anything we desire through creativity and imagination. One can change one's thinking process. Hence, "As a man thinketh so is he." Behavior is reflected from the attitude.

Love is rooted physically in the heart. The heart receives

and gives (the creative and the receptive). It is a continuous gentle flow in harmony. There is no separation. Mankind isolates himself from himself and the universe. We have to learn to obey the laws of nature because the same resides within us. Nature teaches us the laws, the universe is a living being. We all belong and are part of this being, referred to as *God*. To question God is not accepting what is. Life is, the universe is, eternity is. Life is sacred, life always is healthy. Only through our wrong thinking and belief systems do our bodies and minds become unhealthy and die. Fear is the underlying cause of dis-ease both mentally and physically. Since life is rooted in love there is nothing to fear.

In this book, Dolph tries to make as many people as possible aware of their states of health, consciousness, and the acknowledgment of their capabilities to change anything through a continuous learning process and the basic understanding of the laws of life.

Our life is an infinite series of choices requiring constant reunion and reevaluation. In staying receptive and being creative we open ourselves to the experience of life. Only in the experience do we feel we are alive. Instead we are reacting to everything which we call our world.

We have abdicated our power out of fear, out of exaggerated and misunderstood desires, and have therefore collectively created a world of dis-ease, mass destruction through weapons, unprecedented violence and sensationalism, overreaction to outer stimuli, be it drugs, alcohol, sex or television. Through our ignorance and negligence we are supporting a government of corruption and waste. All of this is a reflection of an ill value system which is not responsive to the basic needs and well-being of our society.

Today's society offers and exemplifies poor health, poor education, and poor environment. Man has derived his laws which are not in accordance with the universal laws. Due to mismanagement in this country we are experiencing economic upheaval. On one side there is unparalleled wealth and waste, on the other poverty and death which we consciously support through our apathy, fear and taxes. Yet we like to hide our heads in the sand bemoaning the fact that the air and water is polluted, our food chemical and artificial. Just as our bodies need fresh air, organic food and physical exercise, so does our psyche need beauty, love, rest and music.

Our hospitals are reflections of gross incompetence and stupidity. People are treated as cattle in the fields, and human factor has been forgotten. Man's intelligence and creativity has been underestimated. Many people leave their lives and fate in the hands of ignorance. The body is treated without considering the soul.

In today's medicine people are classified through X-rays and blood tests, and treated with standardized textbook remedies which are at best marginal. The results are in many cases lifetime treatments of one sort or another, surgery from which you may emerge with vital organs, glands, muscles or bones missing. For the sake of health and well-being, drugs are prescribed and injected which leave behind the effect of a nuclear war and disaster upon the body. One has only to survey a physician's desk reference to learn of the harmful possibilities and side effects which exist when one takes various drugs. Then there are such diseases called terminal or schizophrenic; should you be afflicted or at least diagnosed with one or the other you might as well turn yourself in. We have a responsibility toward our well-being and doctors should *not* be blamed if they are not fulfilling the needs of the individual. Live and well-being lies within oneself and can only be well-guided and directed and not subordinated.

It is becoming increasingly clear that humanity must reorganize itself and recognize the basic needs in living and reconstruct and reform intelligently and responsibly a positive change in our society.

We can live healthier lives through education and self-evaluation and learn this process. We must eliminate those forces in society which bleed and destroy us or hamper the quality of life. We need to be honest and sincere as to what is really important. We must recognize and accept that true healing is an educational as well as an evolutionary process. We must redirect and demand an end to all the senseless waste, greed for power, competition, and disrespect for human suffering, when in our very midst the cancer is growing, an epidemic disease which is not understood by those who say they are our benefactors.

We are living within the mind of God and we all are a microcosm of this one aspect. It is time to wake up and accept the endowment of all the great teachings available. Children must grow up and lead responsible lives; we cannot allow more upheaval and havoc to destroy our planet and ourselves.

There will always be thought-mind-spirit. One must never stop; awareness is recognition. There is no new thought or old thought or exceptional events. All events have already happened and have been. In the awareness we experience the event. If aware, the experience teaches to become; when experiencing fully ourselves we become the event, part of the universe already happened, destined to happen and to become. Recognition of that has brought us closer to God-like beings. The universe is the substance of God—is all in perfect flow and union at all times.

Acceptance has to do with the time concept; to be in the now is the experience from which we grow. Time does not exist as we perceive it. We get caught and lost in time.

To question God is not accepting—God is, life is, you are.

Ehlah Pascal

Contents

Acknowledgments

To my wife Ehlah Pascal whose profound influence, intelligence, insight and understanding helped to generate the knowing of the more profound realities of existence. To her persistence in helping to remove the blinders of illusion where during many a night the finer points of philosophy were brought to the light of direct experience; to her infinite patience as I struggled with new ideas and possibilities which to her were perfectly clear but to me were either so nebulous or terrifying, and finally I acknowledge her indomitable love and beauty without which this book would never have been written.

In friendship and respect to Jason, a Qabalistic philosopher and educator, whose understanding and humanity have touched me deeply.

To Dr. Stephen Chang an acupuncturist who explained Taoist philosophy and the principles of yin-yang.

To Jean-Claude, a friend and artist.

To my closest friends and family who have supported me throughout my life.

To the artists of the world who through their efforts continually help to illuminate their fellow man to the beauty and joy of creation.

Song of Change

The world is as secure as an eggshell
And one day it shatters all to pieces

And you don't know how it happened
And you don't know where to go
And you don't know what to do about it
And you don't know how to fall
And you don't know where you're at
And you don't know who you are
And you don't know what is what
And you don't know what we are—

Will there be rebirth again
Will there be much laughter
Will I feel great love in vain
Will I be . . . at all—
Knowing that in time
I'll have changed from life to death
Have I lived at all . . .

The mind always fears
The body demands
But the soul is immortal

Ehlah Pascal

Dedication

To my beloved Ehlah whose wisdom and inspiration brought
forth this book and helped to show me the miracles of life.

Introduction

It was a day of death when I graduated from medical school. I remember vaguely a lot of noise, handshaking, congratulations and excitement around me. What for? I felt so lonely, lost and in a state of confusion and despair. What is happening? Why am I not sharing all this excitement? I realized it was a total loss of direction in terms of my profession. What to do?

I headed west. After drifting around for several months I ended up in San Francisco where I entered into an externship for lack of money and a desire to work.

My life took a radical change when I met Ehlah, who through her own being, knowledge and understanding began to make clear to me the deeper aspects of life and its infinite possibilities. She began to bring light into the darkness of my mind and the process of awakening began. Besides being a philosopher, Ehlah is an experiencer of life, seeing and living life as an artist, aware of life's inherent movements and beauty. Through her example and inspiration as well as being introduced to Qabalistic philosophy (a philosophy of profound insight, love and truth which concerns itself with self-under-standing), it became clear and is becoming increasingly clear that life and man are part of an evolutionary process which is always moving towards greater and greater degrees of consciousness and understanding. And what lies behind the world of appearances, our everyday waking state, which often creates the idea that life and the world is a bad or miserable situation is something which is so profound, so rich, so intelligent, so loving, so beautiful and so supporting that those fortunate beings who have truly seen or felt the deeper aspects of their inner beings have undergone dramatic changes of attitude in regards to nature of life in general.

We must first try to understand and then never forget that our personal selves, our personal mind, are intimately connected to a vast ocean of consciousness which defies intellectual comprehension. Every movement, every breath, every action, every thought is a direct result of the lifeforce working and moving through each and everyone of its creations. And this lifeforce, this intelligence of which we are all aspects, is always working towards its own freedom. This urge for freedom which is synonymous with the urge toward love is the deepest, most profound archetypal desire existing within man.

This love is experienced emotionally as happiness.

The world we live in is a world of our own making. If we do not like it we have the power to change it. Change occurs from within *not* from without. There is nothing wrong with life, it's just our perception of it which creates the illusion that it is not perfect. We need to get our values and priorities straightened out and we need to clear our heads just as we need to clear our water, our air, our food, and our hearts. Our bodies need clean water, healthy food, sunshine and exercise. Our minds or psyche needs *beauty*, silence and cultivation.

We are now moving into the Aquarian age, an age of

love, peace, and harmony and those who understand will let go mentally and physically of those institutions, beliefs and attitudes which oppose man's natural inherent goodness and forestall the inevitable movement toward light and love. It is a time of healing, a time of mutual understanding, and a time of death-rebirth. Man is created in the image of God and if we are all true to ourselves then we must let die those forces which imprison our minds and bodies so that we may truly embrace the concepts of *life, liberty* and the pursuit of happiness.

Amen!!!

1

Basic Philosophy

Who are we? What is our purpose? These are questions which have been pondered by millions of searching minds throughout man's course of existence. They may be answered from various aspects all of which will lead to a basic truth. For instance, it has been said that man is created in the image of God. This implies man's inherent divinity, that He and His Creator are intimately related. To answer these questions with a concept of what God is, lies beyond intellectual understanding. However, it can be seen and experienced in that everything which exists is a manifestation of an unlimited consciousness, directing life power, which expresses itself continuously in an infinite variety of forms and possibilities. Underlying this manifestation is a basic primal energy, a conscious light energy which permeates and sustains all things. There is no thing which exists apart from this conscious infinite energy.

Esoteric philosophy both Eastern and Western agree that *God* is an infinite conscious radiant energy which creates itself out of itself. As it is stated in the *Book of Tokens*.

Meditation

I am
    Without beginning, without end,
    Older than night or day,
Younger than the babe newborn,
    Brighter than light,
    Darker than darkness,
Beyond all things and creatures,
Yet fixed in the heart of everyone.

From me the shining worlds flow forth,
To me all at last return,
Yet to me neither men nor angels
May draw nigh,
For I am known only to myself.

Ever the same is mine inmost being;
Absolutely one, complete, whole, perfect;
            Always itself;
Eternal, infinite, ultimate;
Formless, indivisible, changeless.

Of all existences I am the source,
The continuation, and the end.
    I am the germ
    I am the growth
    I am the decay
All things and creatures I send forth;
I support them while yet they stand without;
And when the dream of separation ends,
I cause their return unto myself.

    I am the Life,
    And the Wheel of the Law,

And the Way that leadeth to the Beyond.
    There is none else.

I am the Fire of Mind
Which divideth itself
Into the Superior and Inferior natures
And putteth on a robe of flesh
To come down.

I am the vital principal of all that is.
Nothing is that does not live,
And of that life I am the source.

As it is written:
    "First the stone,
    Then the plant,
    Then the animal,
    And then the man."
But before the stone, I am the Fire,
Distributed equally in space,
Nowhere absent, filling all
And before the Fire, hidden within it,
I am the pure KNOWING
Whence all forms flow forth.

    Apart from me
    There is neither wisdom,
    Nor knowledge, nor understanding.
Into every state of knowledge do I enter,
Into false knowledge as well as into true,
So that I am not less the ignorance of the deluded
Than the wisdom of the sage.

For what thou callest ignorance and folly
Is my pure knowing,

Imperfectly expressed
Through an uncompleted image
Of my divine perfection.

 Woe unto them
Who condemn these my works unfinished!
Behold, they who presume to judge
Are themselves incomplete.
Through many a fiery trial of sorrow
    Must they pass
Ere the clear beauty of my wisdom
May shine from out their hearts,
    Like unto a light
Burning in a lamp of alabaster.

I am the doer of all.
Nothing moveth but by my power.

Mine is the healing influence
Flowing down from consecrated hands,
Mine the venom of the adder's fang.
    Nothing falleth but by me
And in whatsoever riseth
Mine is the power that lifteth up.

My presence is the substance of all things.
I am the virgin snow on mountain heights;
I am the fruitful loam in valley depths.
I am the gold and silver of the temple vessels,
I am the mire on sandals left by the faithful
    at the temple gate.
See me and regard me equally in all, O Israel,
And thou shalt see indeed.

For seeing thus, shalt thou see, too,

That nothing is, or can be, my antagonist.
   All, and in all
   Shall I fight myself?
What hath power to limit or defeat
The very source of power?

Know then, that all they sense of conflict
Is but the shadow-play of ignorance.
Wait with patience on me, thy Lord,
And in my appointed time
Will I make clear what now is dark,
And show before thee, straight and true
   A path of safety
In the very place where now an abyss of terror
Seems to open at thy feet.

I am the beginning of all beginnings,
Checked by neither time nor space,
Held by no bonds of name or form.
   Present everywhere,
Centering the full perfection
Of mine exhaustless power,
I am thy Lord, O Israel,
And Lord of countless hosts.
Seek me in the Holy of Holies,
In the heart of the true Temple,
On the Holy Mountain
Behold, I am with thee always,
And I never sleep.

I am the Height above all heights.
My descent reacheth likewise below all depths.
Yet I am poised forever between Height and Depth
   In perfect balance.
Consider me under the aspect of ALEPH;

There shalt thou find both Height and Depth
And the path also which joineth them
    For descent and return.

    ALEPH in truth am I,
    The OX of solar fire
Whose radiance lighteth all the world,
Whose life-breath ebbeth and floweth
In creatures great and small,
Whose power taketh form
In all the acts of men, of beasts, of plants,
Yea, and of things which seem inanimate, as well.

ALEPH am I, the patient burden-bearer,
Strong to carry the heavy load of the manifest.
ALEPH am I, the Eternal Worker,
By whose might all fields are tilled,
And from whose life all seeds
Derive their growth and increase.

    ALEPH am I,
    The First and the Root.
From mine unfathomable Will
The universe hath its beginning.
In my boundless Wisdom
Are the types and patterns of all things.

    Before all worlds I WAS;
    In all worlds I AM;
And when worlds are but a memory,
    I SHALL BE.

From a scientific point of view, we have come to know that
man is composed of atoms and electrons vibrating at a particular frequency. The substance of every atom is identical
with what is sometimes called "radiant energy," "light,"

"electromagnetism." These are different names for one thing. We can view ourselves as *light* in a particular form which is contained within the context of a space-time continuum and held together by the forces of gravity.

Since all substance is composed of similar building blocks—that is, atomic and subatomic particles at various stages of evolution—we may assume that everything is alive and that form is but a reflection of vibration and energy.

The concept of soul or spirit or consciousness is subjective and cannot be scientifically proven, however, theoretical physics is moving closer and closer to a unifying theory of consciousness based on the principles of pulsatile energy. Inherent within all substance is a pulsating life-force. All life is in this state of pulsation, moving through states of contraction and expansion. All life exhibits this rhythm, the heart of course being the most notable example.

It is interesting to note here the relationship between science (physics) and religious philosophy (metaphysics). When Jesus said, "I am the light of the world," he was stating a scientific fact; in Qabalistic philosophy that light is *Ensophor*, the limitless light or no-thing from which all things are derived. Science uses the measure of light as the one absolute, the measure by which all other things are measured. Einstein's theory of relativity established that all our measurements are imperfect for they are measurements of relationships between the same things—light or electromagnetic radiation. We are units of light-energy, controlled and directed through will or desire (life power).

The development of the atomic and hydrogen bombs unequivocally showed that inherent within "things" are enormous powers which may be released. From a symbolic point of view the unleashing of the atomic bomb may be seen as the realization of man's infinite potential. We are reservoirs of enormous creative energy which are as yet unrealized—and poorly controlled.

While the atom bomb unveiled the limitless power of the

universe, the psychedelic age unveiled the profundity and power of the human psyche. Man learned (as some men have always known) that existence may be experienced in various states of consciousness and that *reality* is not a fixed perception. Man also came to know in a very exact, profound way that his beliefs and attitudes create an immediate reality. The subconscious is always receptive to suggestion and the suggestion is experienced as reality, relative to the nature of the suggestion. It appears that when one uses a consciousness altering substance he experiences an aspect of his subconscious mind.

Human beings have had extraordinary ranges of experience, experiences of union with the self or the creative intelligence in which many realized that *they* and *it* were aspects of the same thing. Subject-object relationships fell apart. Many came to know that God cannot be personified and that the only reality is light energy which may take an infinite variety of forms be it music, color, sounds, other beings, other worlds . . . Experience became a Gestalt of movement, feeling, ecstasy (freedom), ever changing—ever moving, without beginning—without end.

We learned that consciousness may expand beyond physicality and that we can indeed explore the *mind* of which we are intimately a part. We also came to know that the cosmos contains positive and negative forces, and while bliss, light and ecstasy were desirable states, the opposite poles exist as well where fears and anxieties are projected and experienced. Within our subconscious mind is not only a perfect record of this life's experience but also a record of the history of man. This aspect of our mind has been appropriately described by Carl Jung as the *collective unconscious*.

The ego or personality is one aspect of our subconcious. This aspect of our "beingness" is supported by and dependent upon the creative aspect of mind which is the self or higher self. However, as long as we identify strictly with the physical nature or ego-drives of our being then we are caught within self-imposed limitations and illusions. The self is infinite, boundless and beyond time; the body is a vehicle, an expression of the self.

We are beginning to recognize the possibility that life on earth can be a joyous, growing, creative experience and that life is a process of evolution "moving" toward greater perception, awareness and understanding. Getting there is no more important than *being here*; the illusion of "Heaven" and "Hell" has been irrevocably shattered as we recognize that in some way or other we create our own reality through our perception and attitude.

Using our greater awareness, we now know that morality is a fixed, stagnant set of beliefs imposed by others as to how one should behave, act and think. We consciously realize that each and every individual has within himself the ability to know his own personal truth and gain control of his own life. Many of us now hold the firm belief that the universe or cosmos is a joyous, creative, expanding entity derived from thought filled with countless other personalities unified consciously or unconsciously through love.

As man is a part of nature, we are subject to universal laws, the same universal laws which govern nature. It is man's deepest desire to seek balance, to attain peace and harmony within the universe in which we find ourselves. Man is his own universe, he is the microcosm within the macrocosm. As man observes nature he is in reality observing aspects of himself. We may come to know the constancy of change, the movements of the seasons, the ebb and flow of emotions; the cyclic periodic rhythms in nature which are reflected within man. We are continuously influenced by subtle forces, be they astrological, natural, environmental, or personal. Everything affects everything else.

It is our inability to work within periodicity and cycles that causes much of the difficulty in the use and misuse of our energies, particularly the sublimating or excessive expression of the sexual urge both through physical expression and fantasy. This failure to live by the "law of periodicity" (being true to ourselves) and the relative inability to subordinate the various needs and appetities to cyclic control is the challenge of man. It is also this failure of control which is one of the major causes of disease.

We are our own ecological system maintaining itself in a state of dynamic equilibrium through subconscious and self-conscious control of biofeedback mechanisms. In states of relative calm or relaxation, the body functions automatically under the control of the subconscious mind, maintaining the necessary homeostatic mechanisms necessary for the maintenance of life. In states of fight or flight (fear or anxiety) the organism elaborates a myriad of hormones to increase sugar production, increase the heart rate, elevate the metabolism. Thus, it is the manner in which we experience our reality which determines the relative health of our bodies. In other words, if an individual is consistently angry, fearful or hateful his body will in a real way reflect these negative, painful emotions.

Our emotions are translated from thought feelings (energy) into biophysical impulses carried down the spinal cord. The autonomic nervous system is connected to the higher cortical regions of the brain and innervates via its sympathetic and parasympathetic components the various glands, blood vessels, organs and tissues of the body. This relationship is the basis of psychosomatic medicine.

Fear is a product of the mind and fear may be abolished by changing one's behavior and/or thinking patterns. In other words, we start to consciously give different suggestions to ourselves which are experienced as different emotions—our attitudes and beliefs create our state of health.

We need to recognize that energy follows thought. Our bodies (I include the brain as well) are but vehicles of expression of the "higher self" or "self." Every moment of our waking consciousness is motivated and conditioned by some type of *desire*. Our desire is a product of internal and external factors and forces. It is conditioned by our educational system, parents, peers, TV, newspapers or whatever imprints in our subconscious. As children we are vulnerable to an infinite variety of suggestions.

Thus, we may view ourselves as a biocomputer filled with innumerable programs fed to us consciously and subconsciously throughout our impressionable years—that time where we are not able to consciously discriminate what we choose to believe as true or not true. These programs create our habit patterns of behavior which operate on a subconscious level. The subconscious mind is always amenable to suggestion.

The degree to which we are conscious, that is the degree to which we know what we are doing and why we are doing it, is the degree to which we are able to think for ourselves and perceive our personal reality. All too often our actions and desires are in deep conflict with our true desires. We have been consistently told what we need to be healthy and happy, not realizing that we are able to determine this for ourselves. The mass mind has created the tremendous impulse in this country for materialism and a hectic pace of life. There is nothing wrong with "materialism" in itself, however, when it becomes the reason for being and the driving, motivating force in a person's life then we are out of touch; the nature of man is both spiritual and physical.

The unconscious or self-conscious man sees himself as a body devoid of spirit, reacting, always attempting to fulfill ego-needs—sex, food, sensation, power, fame, or whatever. Man in his isolation sees himself apart from everything else —he is not tuned into himself or his environment and expressions such as love, art, compassion, sensitivity are but abstractions. He follows a false messiah of endless addictions which continuously create further addicted behavior which leads to dissatisfaction, frustration, boredom, anger, and distraction.

Within everyone lies the potential to experience self as an intimate part of the cosmos of which they are a unique extension. The unconscious man has not awakened to the creative potential which lies within him. He sees the world as a threat, as a political struggle of *Us* vs. *Them*; blind to the reality that *Us* is *Them* in a very real way, and the horrors which exist in the world are but the collective anxieties and projected fears of similar-minded individuals.

Man reflects the limitations and suffering of over-identification with the body which we define as the *ego*. The ego is not something to be killed or destroyed; it is to be tamed and controlled through judicious self-discipline and self- observation.

It is through the senses, that we may experience our spirituality. Our desires create our reality and if they are not in keeping with universal law then we find ourselves in conflict and disease. Through love and the understanding of the emotions one can begin to control the ego. *We reap what we sow* and if we don't like the reality that is formed we have the power to change it. This is a process of self-understanding and it entails trial and error. We learn through experience and the experience becomes our feedback if consciously examined. The problem is in reconditioning the way we think; we must learn to reject or no longer energize those false attitudes and beliefs which create conflict and inner turmoil.

We get help in our struggle to clear and open the mind because this Life. of which we are all a part is a collective working toward Its total liberation. We experience this as a raising of our individual consciousness. Collectively our higher energies can and will in time balance and calm the irrational turbulence of the ego-driven mind. This will only occur, however, when we open ourselves to these energies;

we focus our attention upon something greater than ourselves; we begin to break through resistances which prevent
or block the free flow of energy.

It is love-energy (grace) which sustains us and it may be
received and transmitted in various ways. Man's struggle is
basically that of learning to accept love which is given unconditionally. It is there at all times, but the clouds of our
negative emotions and programming prevent this from happening. We do not permit ourselves the pleasure of opening
up to the possibility of unconditional love. We close it off —
we become uptight.

We hurt, we suffer, we become *dis*-eased because the
healing energies are not permitted to flow throughout the
body. As love and energy flow through our corporeal being
we experience peace, harmony and knowingness; we experience that all our trials and processes have been to teach us to
experience just this.

Once we come to accept the flow of energy, we become
aware of the rhythm and flow of the universe. As we learn to
become receivers and transmitters of energy we experience
greater degrees of joy, happiness and creativity. To withhold
this energy or love is to create blocks within ourselves which
in time manifest themselves as *dis*-ease, physical or mental.
Thus, the body is an exquisitely sensitive *feedback* mechanism which continually communicates our emotions through
feelings.

Bodily health is maintained through the *subconscious
mind*. All disease processes have their origins within the
realm of the mind: healthy mind, healthy body. The higher
energies emanating through us control the lower forces
(instinctual animal drives) and the change that then occurs is
a raising of consciousness. (The science of alchemy actually
deals with the trasmutation of the personality and the moving from one energy state to another.) Once we recognize
that we can reprogram our subconscious mind via self-con-

scious suggestion we are able to consciously control our own evolution.

Dis-ease may be seen as the failure of the physical body to bring in these higher energies. Whether we fail and to what extent we fail is dependent upon our particular point in evolution as reflected in our personal awareness and self-knowledge.

Evolution is change in process, and as we are intimately a part of the universe we need to move with the flow of the universe. To resist this change is to swim upstream against the current. This upstream struggle is really a struggle against ourselves.

The real self, our deepest truest nature, knows and understands itself perfectly, and is moving within the energy flow. The ego, the sense of personal identity, believes itself to be the doer and mover of the universe and therefore is caught in an illusion of separateness which creates the sense of isolation, fear and anxiety that is the precursor of disease. Our real purpose in life is to consciously align ourselves with ourselves remebering always that the cosmos (collective consciousness) is always working to liberate and free itself. Or, in a religious idiom, divine grace is always at our disposal, we only have to be receptive to it.

The mind and attitudes of the individual is changed through the self working through subconscious mental activity. The resultant change is the subjective feelings of increased energy, well-being and happiness. This process of evolution is essentially a reawakening process in which we are led out of darkness and illusion into the light of understanding.

As we strive to gain conscious control of our ego state, we are moving toward a balance of negative and positive energies. The Taoist concept of this balance is reflected as the Yin-Yang:

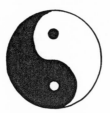

The negative forces interacting with the positive energies creating a dynamic equilibrium expressed as the middle way.

The negative aspect is considered the feminine and the positive aspect is the masculine. The positive-negative polarities represent self-conscious/man and subconscious/woman—this is the *anima* and *animus* in Jungian terminology. The *Shiva-Shakti* principle in Hinduism.

The balancing of these "lower" forces with the "higher" forces may be represented symbolically in Western terms.

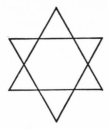

The Star of David is symbolic of the integration of both the conscious (masculine) and subconscious (female) aspect of personality. This integration is experienced as Love.

Our life's purpose, consciously or unconsciously, is directed toward the establishment of this dynamic equilibrium. This impetus toward self-understanding is not based on ego-drives but on the intense desire of the self to re-unite with itself.

What evidence today do we have that these energies really exist within and outside of ourselves and that we really are more than complex biological machines? The vital life energy which supports and sustains and permeates all things has been given many names. The Hebrews called it *ruach*; the Hindus called it *prana*, the Greeks *pneuma*, the Latins *spiritus*, the Chinese *chi*.

The Oriental systems of medicine have known and understood the reality of these energy currents for over 5,000 years. They compose the meridian system which is the basis of acupuncture. These energy conduits are in communication with the skin and conduct energy to various organ systems. Dis-ease or pain is considered within the concept of Chinese medical philosophy to be a result of an unequal distribution of the flow of energy. *Imbalance* and *disease* are synonymous and the factor responsible for such a situation is either too much energy or too little energy.

The Tibetan Buddhists referred to these meridian currents as *niduses* and were of like mind as regards to the cause of disease manifestation. The ancients understood how these energy currents flow and bathe the entire body in a rhythmic, cyclic fashion.

The pioneering work in Kirlian photography provides convincing evidence that human beings are surrounded by and bathed in an aura of electromagnetic energy exerting its influence into the environs.

The understanding of the body as a unity is part of Eastern medicine which is based upon deep philosophic insight. It is implied that if the organism is flowing, expressive, creative and hence alive it does not get sick; it is following its own path and recognizes the unity and diversity of all that is.

What we are witnessing today is a universal change of self-image. Man is beginning to understand in a conscious way what he has always known about himself, that we are an inherent part of the cosmos, in continuous communication with it, and that we possess free-will (not a personal will as much as a primal will acting through the agency of personality).

Only our lack of exploration of ourselves and abdication of responsibility to others keeps us from consciously experiencing the truth. The life-force inherent within and shared by all of us must be expressed and manifested. This is progressive and cannot be stopped, it is an inexorable movement greater than any one man. It is life, it is the Tao, and as expanding, evolving beings each and every one of us is trying to comprehend and experience this awesome truth. It is my firm belief that the nature of man is good and the purpose of our existence is to experience love, peace, joy, happiness and goodwill.

The key to life and health is creativity, spontaneity, joy, reasonableness, laughter and a healthy self-image. We should rejoice in the knowledge that we are, always have been and always will be.

2

Human Sexuality and Sexual Energy

There is probably no other area of human affairs which so readily presents the problems and potentials of the human experience as does human sexuality. Human sexuality must be examined from the perspective of balance: How do repression and excessive sexual desire create pathology in the human being? How does love—the harmonizing force which brings stability, resonance and harmony—allow human beings to flow through life?

There is no more compelling desire within the human heart than for freedom and the desire of union with oneself and with another. It is in the realm of human sexuality and sensuality that these intense, archetypal desires may be manifested. To deny the sensuality inherent in our biological nature is to deny our reality.

Many of us are caught in a nasty dualism brought about by our conditioning and the intellectualization of our humanness. The average person today has as his greatest longing the expression of his love energy. Lovemaking implies a creative act, a *desire* to initiate an action. It is an act which requires attention to detail, patience, a desire to please another person. Lovemaking is a process to give and take, a sharing and cycling of mutual energies, a breaking down or breaking through of resistances (inhibitions) to feelings, to touching, to individual expression. Lovemaking is an art. The act is the primordial creative expression of the universe. The desire of union is as strong a drive in nature as exists.

Our pain very often can be seen as a resistance or denial of this basic truth. The fear associated with the sex act is well-known and understood. Embarrassment, lack of self-confidence, fear of failure, fear of not pleasing, are all emotions which are experienced by people. However, the denial of our natural feelings, the suppression of these tendencies creates enormous imbalances within the human psyche and body. This conflict manifests itself as anxiety. Blocked emotions have a pronounced effect upon the autonomic nervous system as well as the skeletal musculature of the body.

Real growth and spiritual fulfillment may be learned and appreciated through our sexuality. The body and its sensations allow us to be conscious of "being." The body needs touching, feeling and movement to experience itself. In lovemaking resonance and harmony are possible; this is a mind-body phenomenon that allows us the possibility of experiencing intense transcending feelings. The achievement of total and complete orgasm is actualized by the capacity for surrender to the flow of biological energy without any inhibition.

The range of human experience in regards to pleasure and sensation in the sexual act is legion. Tantra, the Indian cult of ecstasy, portends that through sexual rituals and meditations one may attain spiritual insight and liberation. We can find ourselves in another; we can lose our feelings of alienation and loneliness; we can experience joy and transcend to ecstatic levels of consciousness. All these are very real possibilities. The sexual act reflects the basic pulsation of the universe: the building up (tension), the discharge of energy (orgasm), relaxation; then the cycle repeats itself.

We can "die" to ourselves in the lovemaking process; we intuitively understand this and letting go is something we all desire yet find so difficult to do. We become cynical, except for those who have experienced truly exalted feelings and know that love is not an abstraction but an experience which transcends words and is totally subjective. It moves beyond the rational, intellectual mind which incessantly tries to measure and explain what love is. It is a key to our well-being and happiness. It is pure folly to deny our essential sexual nature and it is dangerous to block the attendant desire for contact and union. Most, if not all, of man's difficulties revolve around ambivalent feelings about his sexuality. Anxiety neurosis and depressive episodes are often reflections of sexual imbalance and decreased energy states. Anger and self-hatred can be traced to our inability to share with and communicate our energies to another human being.

Love is as essential to our biologic survival as is food and water. The universe sustains and is sustained by this process and as we are a microcosm within a macrocosm then we should partake of what is available and possible. The male and female are opposite yet complementary aspects of the unity. Each can exist by itself and sustain itself, of course, but united there is recognition that nothing exists that is not an expression of love. This is not to say that we are lost in an eternal embrace—we come together, we flow apart only to come together again. This contraction-expansion, attraction-repulsion, tension-relaxation is a universal rhythm. We need *only* surrender ourselves to our natural inherent rhythms to understand this. It is the conditioning, cultural taboos, overemphasis on objective materialistic reality which imposes itself and works against our natural self.

Opposite to those who partake in the delight of tantric practice lie the individuals who are totally ego-bound, full of inhibition, viewing the sexual act as a release of tension—a mutual masturbation of sorts. This attitude and mode of behavior denies the unity of the act and only creates frustration, bitterness and a feeling of emptiness. Most people fall somewhere between these two polarities.

There is another element which espouses asceticism. The concept being that denial of the body may allow the individual to transcend his biological nature and center his attention on "spiritual matters." It is a difficult path, fraught with struggle and deep-seated conflict, particularly in young people.

Life is a series of choicies; it is not for us to criticize others; however, to deny the physical aspect of what we are is to deny a major aspect of the human experience. As we age and our sexual passions abate, then our consciousness may reflect upon itself and turn away from the material aspect and concentrate and explore the realms of the subconsicous.

For a couple to indulge in passionate, fulfilling lovemaking we must understand the process of "getting to know" each other. The advantage of bond relationships as in marriage is that it creates a commitment to each other. This commitment if honestly fulfilled frees the individuals from sexual fantasy and continual projections of sexual energy onto others. We may come to see other people as people rather than sex objects to be manipulated and used. It allows a healthy, balanced sexuality to unfold and there is no pressure to have continuous, consuming affairs based solely on physical attraction.

A couple may come to understand that lovemaking need not involve genital union. A loving couple may find that massage, caressing and embracing will suffice. This removes a tremendous pressure off each other as there is no longer a need to perform well. The relationship becomes more flowing and natural if there is a deep commitment between the couple to keep the relationship growing in all ways.

In any relationship we need to see and recognize that we are involving not two identities but four. We are dealing with incessant yet subtle changes day to day and need to understand that the personality is capable of acting out an impressive array of characters. We are not married to just one person so to speak; we are multi-dimensional personalities and therein lies the freshness and renewing aspect of any long-term relationship. Within the subconscious reside the feminine and masculine aspects. In esoteric psychology these aspects are termed the *receptive* and *creative* aspects, or in Jungian terms the *anima* and *animus*. These elements need to be harmonized and recognized within the individual, this is a process of conscious evolution and learning the essence of what we are. Therefore, we may see the fulfilling sexual act as a culmination of self-knowledge and understanding. We no longer identify with the body but recognize and feel that the higher self is directing and manifesting the action.

Anxiety, fear, inhibition create obstacles to this fulfillment and it is for this reason that the proper setting should be created to help facilitate lovemaking. Expectation, obligation, previsualization, submissiveness and other ego drives impede the actualization and flowing of somatic and psychic energy. Love creates a harmonic resonance between the opposites (male and female) and frees the consciousness of the individual allowing us to explore the collective consciousness. Time and space collapse and our entire attention and concentration is residing in the eternal now. It is in this space that one intuitively recognizes the enormity that "you" is "me" and "me" is "you."

The longer the process is continued the greater the excitation and tension which is created—the process rather than the product is the motivation. The orgasm or climax directs a rush of energy down through the spine where it flows throughout the entire nervous system; also the voluntary muscular system moves through the same process of tension (excitation) and relaxation. Thus, the entire organism is bathed in a rush of light and healing energy. We subconsciously know this and it may explain the enormity of the sexual drive in humans as well as in other animals. It is a replication of the pulse of the universe and our chance to tune into and be resonant with the universal energies.

Man as all other animals is subject to basic patterns of ebb and flow. We have our "high" and our "low" periods. As we tune into our feelings and cycles we know and recognize the building of our sexual energies. If we learn to follow our rhythms then we are living within our *Tao*. However, we possess free will and through our creative intelligence and directed effort we may circumvent the natural oncoming feelings and indulge and impose our own schedule, thereby creating a block to the natural flow of energy.

Implicit in trying to attain sexual satisfaction is the recognition that a subtle, flexible body capable of smooth coordinated movement facilitates the action. To lead healthy sexually exciting lives we must realize that the body must be taken care of. Our bodies are the temples of our souls and our bodies are creative expressions of our higher energies.

We have the energy which drives and motivates us through our life and we witness continuously the squandering and misdirection of it. Balance requires choice and conscious direction of energy. Our attitudes, values and priorities will move us either in the direction of a harmonizing relationship or perhaps into various subtle ego-games where we will find ourselves putting most of our energy into loner-games or ego-gratification. This is our choice. However, by placing our emphasis upon these games, we divest ourselves from ourselves. A relationship between two people takes constant work and energy to sustain it.

There has been much written today about the act of masturbation. For our purposes, excessive masturbation is considered counter-productive in that it is a needless, undi-

rected depletion of energy stores. In Chinese medical philosophy the strength and essence of a man resides within his
germinal essence, his semen. To waste and deplete this continuously lowers the total energy of the organism. Sex is but
one aspect of life within our natural rhythm.

It appears that Western man is addicted to sex as he is to
food and spends most of his time either fantasizing about it or
engaged in superficial relationships which bring little satisfaction. The Taoist state that one need not ejaculate during
the sex act and that orgasm and pleasure may be attained
without ejaculation. The idea is that the male and female
bring each other up to a point of sexual excitement and tension and play on the edges of this excitement realizing that
when the male ejaculates the sexual pleasure abates. This, of
course, takes tremendous self-discipline and work; the art of
Tantra is based primarily on similar concepts.

If we over masturbate or ejaculate then we deplete our
energy store and time is needed to reestablish our potency.
Interestingly enough the Bible has a subtle refrain against
tampering with our sexual energies—"cast not your seed
upon the ground"—there are many interpretations of this
and it may be seen in a moralistic context, however I feel the
teachings of the Bible are consistent with the concepts of
energy transfer and energy flow.

Inherent in Taoist concepts as well is the implicit idea
that men and women may remain sexually active well into
their later years—70s, 80s and 90s. The pace of life and
frenetic activity of Western culture lends itself to an early
burning out period and we do not recognize the possibility
that we can live our lives to a much greater duration. The
high incident of benign prostatic hypertrophy and prostatic
cancer appears to me to be intimately related to a premature
cessation of sexual activity. It is a rule of nature that that
which is not utilized or exercised will in time stagnate and
die.

Man's most difficult and challenging problem revolves around his sexual nature and the effective control of his sexual energies. The middle way, a balanced approach to sexual life that is neither repression nor excess will add to the flow and rhythm of our lives as well as creating tremendous gratification and pleasure. Once we recognize that our bodies need stimulation and movement, then we are more apt to try to learn more about our true selves. Communication, that is the meaningful interchange of energy, is essential to our well-being. Sexual boredom often occurs because a couple cannot or will not use their imaginations and experiment with different positions and techniques.

The sexual act and the expression of our natural sensuality can be one path to self-realization. There is perhaps no other area of human endeavor where more has been written or discussed. The topic is filled with controversy and as always we can only know the truth for ourselves by learning through our own direct experience. We need to break through our stifling conditioning and tune into our natural rhythms and pulsations and act accordingly.

3

Nutrition

There is an extraordinary number of misconceptions and controversy about the importance of food and there probably is no area of health where there is so much experimentation. We are all genetically unique, with our own unique metabolic processes. What is beneficial and helpful for one individual may not necessarily be the best thing for another. There is so much introspection, fear and anxiety about what constitutes wholesome food that the negative emotions in themselves create what we are trying to prevent—*dis*-ease.

The one persistent fact that has come from research of cultures noted for their longevity is that these people do not overeat and maintain themselves well on a high-carbohydrate, low-animal protein diet. There are always exceptions to every rule and there will always be individuals who break every rule as to what one should or should not eat and yet enjoy relatively good health. The concept I want to convey is that it is not only what you eat but how you eat it; how it is served and with whom you eat.

The French and Chinese put tremendous emphasis upon varieties of food and their cuisine is a refined art and certainly one of life's great delights. On the other hand, the American style of eating has been caricatured; the emphasis is not so much what you eat but how much you can eat and how fast you can eat it. It is widely felt that the quality of food which is eaten today in the United States is of low quality, that is to say it is adulterated with antibiotics, preservatives, and growth hormones all of which have a definite effect upon our systems. This low quality food (poor nutritional value) lends itself to over-comsumption because the body still is not receiving adequate nutrition. (Over-eating of course is often a sublimation for a repressed sexual drive and is but a manifestation of anxiety.)

Over-comsumption of food is harmful for a variety of reasons. First of all, by consuming large quantities of food we put an unnecessary demand upon the body's digestive system. The body needs energy to digest large quantities of food, for a great deal of work must be done to assimilate it. It is a paradox: We eat food to give us energy and yet in the process of over-eating we expend large amounts of energy to supply our needs. Thus, we can see the creation of a vicious circle. It is interesting to observe people who are on this treadmill, constantly nibbling and feeding. They are addicted to food. It has been said that you can determine the character of a person by how he eats. The gluttonous, ravaging habit may be an indication of extreme anxiety and tension. It may also be a sign that the body is experiencing "starvation amidst plenty," since it is the *quality* of food which satiates and regulates the appetite center of the brin. Eating for many people is a compulsion, the roots of which lie within our conditioning and feeding habits as young children. Eating habits are an important key to self-mastery in that they readily point out the unconscious behavior patterns within us. By careful attention to what we eat and why we eat we can re-learn the condition where real hunger stems from the body and not from neurotic and compulsive behavior.

Our conditioning and life style have completely upset

our natural feeding rhythms. We are inclined to believe that three meals a day are necessary; we constantly find ourselves in situations of either feast or famine to regulate our weight. When we really do enjoy a good meal we punish ourselves and feel guilty about it because we broke our diets. This constant oscillating between imposed desire and basic bodily needs creates emotional and physiological turmoil. It is but another manifestation of imbalance. However, we have the power, if we care to recognize it, to re-establish our *own* basic equilibrium. This requires caring, observation and sensitivity to oneself.

There has been a tremendous growing awareness today in America of how our food supply has been contaminated, adulterated, chemicalized and even poisoned. This has created severe anxiety—real or imagined—and a counter-reaction directed against the food producers of this nation. This awareness of and preoccupation with what we ingest is a healthy movement and will create, through supply and demand, alternate food markets and hopefully a greater sensitivity within the corporate structure which in the past has been totally production and profit motivated. Well, they no doubt eat the same food they sell.

The food business is but another manifestation of our cultural imperatives and priorities. We are becoming increasingly aware that our food chain is in serious jeopardy. We are also aware that much of the soil has been over-farmed and we continue to violate the natural law that tells us we must put back what we take out.

It would be well to note here there are interesting alternatives to the way things are being done currently and one of the more hopeful concepts in horticulture involves the French/Biodynamic intensive farming which restores and respects the natural rhythm and cycles of nature.

The Biodynamic/French intensive method of horticulture is a quiet, vitally alive art of organic gardening which relinks man with the whole universe around him—a universe in which each of us is an interwoven part of the whole. Man finds his place by relating and cooperating in harmony with the sun, air, rain, soil, moon, insects, plants, and animals rather than attempting to dominate them.

The Biodynamic/French intensive method is a combination of two forms of horticulture begun in Europe during the late 1800s and early 1900s. French intensive techniques were developed in the 1890s on two acres of land. Crops were grown on an 18" depth of horse manure, a fertilizer which was readily available. The crops were grown so close to each other that when the plants were mature their leaves would barely touch. The close spacing provided a miniclimate and a living mulch which reduced weed growth and helped hold moisture in the soil. During the winter glass jars were placed over seedlings to give them an early start. The gardeners grew nine crops each year and even grew melons during the winter.

The Biodynamic techniques were developed by Rudolf Steiner, Austrian philosopher and educator in the early 1920s. Noting a decline in the nutritive value and yields of crops in Europe, Steiner traced the cause to the use of the newly introduced inorganic, chemical fertilizers and pesticides. An increase was also noticed in the number of crops affected by disease and insect problems.

Steiner returned to the more gentle, diverse and balanced diets of organic fertilizers as a cure for the ills brought on by inorganic chemical fertilizations. He initiated a movement to scientifically explore the relationship which plants have with each other. From centuries of farmer experience and from tests, it has been determined that flowers, herbs and weeds can minimize insect attacks on plants.

The Biodynamic method brought back raised planting

beds. Two thousand years ago, the Greeks noticed that plant life thrives in landslides. The loose soil allows air, moisture, warmth, nutrients, and roots to properly penetrate the soil.

Sometime between the 1920s and the 1960s, Alan Chadwick, an Englishman, combined the Biodynamic techniques and the French intensive techniques into the Biodynamic/ French intensive method. Mr. Chadwick brought the method to the four-acre student organic garden at the University of California, Santa Cruz, in the 1960s.

The site he developed at Santa Cruz was on the side of a hill with a poor clay soil. The original barren soil was made fertile through extensive use of compost, with its life-giving humus. The humus produced a healthy soil that grew healthy plants less susceptible to disease and insect attacks. The result was beautiful flowers with exquisite fragrances and tasty vegetables of high quality.

This process has demonstrated incredibly high yields of high quality vegetables using minimal ground and organic substances for nutriment. Initial research seems to indicate that "this method produces an average of four times more vegetables/acre than the amount grown by farmers using mechanical and chemical agricultural techniques. This method also appears to use half the water and 1% the energy consumed by commercial agriculture, per pound of vegetable grown. The flavor of the vegetables is usually excellent and there are indications that their nutritive value may be higher. The implications of this method are revolutionary not only because they free up anxiety about a continuing food source but break man's dependence upon artificial fertilizers and technology ... "

Atherosclerosis and coronary heart disease is a national epidemic. Of the approximately 650,000 coronary deaths in the U.S. in 1970 about 175,000 occurred in people aged 35 to 64. For every fatal event at least one, more likely two, major nonfatal ones occurred. Atherosclerosis is a process which leads to hardening, occulsion or weakening of the arteries thereby reducing the blood flow to the tissues. The fundamental lesion of this process is the atheroma which is a discrete plaque arising in the intima of the artery and having a predilection for areas of tortuosity and turbulence of blood flow.

Autopsy studies done on the young Americans killed in Vietnam reconfirmed what was found among the American dead in the Korean War. These men already showed atherosclerotic changes within the major blood vessels of the body and we can correlate this now with the ever-increasingly early onset of myocardial infarctions seen in this country. What initiates this process?

We may attribute this disease to many factors all of which create a decreased oxygen flow at the cellular level along with a poisoning of the internal milieu of cell with interference of the internal respiratory processes of the cell. As each cell is truly a universe unto itself living within the body of a still greater and yet interdependent universe, it is totally dependent upon a continual source of oxygen and nutrients to supply it so that it may remain metabolically active and hence do its work. The cell is a perfectly balanced ecosystem where the forces of anabolism and catabolism are ongoing continual processes. Building up—breaking down; creation—destruction; assimilation—elimination. If the cells internal or external milieu is compromised or poisoned one experiences inefficiency of the cellular respiratory system with a resultant internal acidosis. If this state is prolonged and toxic waste materials are not removed and detoxified then cell death ensues. This is true of all cells. Disease and pathology refect different sites of a similar living process.

The major factors which epidemological studies have indicated to be probable causes of atherosclerosis are:

1. Overconsumption of food, particularly fats and proteins.

2. Lack of exercise.
3. Stress and anxiety.
4. Exposure to environmental pollutants, particularly heavy metals such as lead, mercury, cadmium, and silenium.

Pathogenesis of Atherosclerosis: Atherosclerosis is the result of a focal intimal thickening with various amounts of subendothelial lipid deposits along with deformation and fragmentation of the internal elastic membrane. This is followed by endothelial proliferation. This cellular injury is due primarily to ischemic factors as well as local cellular poisoning of the respiratory enzyme systems of the cells due to chronic exposure and ingestion of heavy metals such as mercury, lead, silenium and cadmium. Known cellular poisons such as lead and cyanide are extremely toxic to the nervous system and will in minute doses (particularly cyanide) create cessation of cellular respiration and hence death. These heavy metals are found in the polluted air we breath, the food we ingest and the cigarette smoke we inhale. The body has natural detoxifying powers, however, if it is continually stressed and insulted like any other machine it will eventually break down.

The delicate, incredibly complex, cellular reactions occurring moment to moment within the cell are catalyzed by enzymes and work in conjunction with trace minerals and vitamins to create heat and energy. If we continually insult this delicate system with poisons then we are jeopardizing the integrity of the cell. The cell literally becomes sick and is not able to efficiently carry out its own natural regenerative process and hence the balance between assimilation and elimination is disrupted. Not only is the internal environment with the cell damaged but the transport mechanism of life-giving oxygen is compromised because of spasm of the surrounding blood vessels themselves. Thus a vicious cycle is established. These waste products and toxins are irritating to the nervous system and disrupt the autonomic nervous system creating

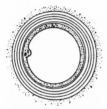

Deposits of lipid
begin to form
beneath the inner
lining of the artery.

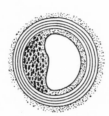

Increase in tissue
cause by lipid
deposits.

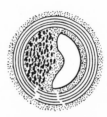

Capillaries begin
to form in tissue
beneath lining.

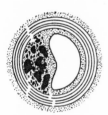

Deposits of lime
salts form in
tissue.

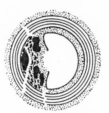

Death of tissue
near inner lining
and ulceration.

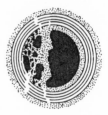

Formation of a
blood clot
blocking the
artery—
thrombosis.

Atheriosclerosis

further alternations of blood flow. Everything effects everything else. The integrity of the cell is disrupted and its cellular contents leak out. We see this microscopically as a build-up within the atheroma of lipids, cholesterol, and calcium. These intracellular materials irritate the environment leading to an attempt to seal off and heal the area. This leads to fibrosis and calcification which leads to necorsis, ulceration, and eventual thrombosis. When the integrity of the endothelial cells have been damaged a scarring process occurs whereby the natural elasticity of the vessel wall is lost and is replaced by relatively inelastic materials.

The fact that atherosclerotic vascular disease is a result of our cultural experience is best exemplified by a remarkable epidemological study carried out among the Bantu nation in Africa. This nation-tribe comprises approximately 50 million people. Atherosclerotic heart disease is virtually absent. These people also show no evidence of colonic carcinoma, hemorrhoids, diverticular disease or hiatal hernias. They live on a high carbohydrate (fruits and vegetables), low fat, low protein diet. They also are not exposed to the stresses and strains of modern industrial society. They are remarkably healthy people whose lives are simple and relaxed. The incidence of heart disease in the Orient is also minor as compared to this country. Diet obviously is an extremely important factor as well as the life style and attitudes.

What can we do now to prevent and reverse this trend which inflicts an incaluable cost in pain and suffering in our society? The answer lies in prevention. It is incumbent upon the medical profession to re-educate itself and thereby instruct and educate the people regarding the real dangers of over-consumption and lack of exercise. Also the medical profession and the people must become more politically aware and demand an end to the poisoning and destruction of the biosphere. Human ecology is intimately related to the ecology of the environment. Man is a part of nature. If we poison and disrupt the ecosystem of the earth we are poisoning and disrupting ourselves. As we detoxify and clean up the earth we are in a real sense purifying and detoxifying ourselves. This is our collective responsibility!

A promising advance in helping to speed up the detoxification process was recently announced at a recent meeting of the orthomelecular medical society. It has been shown both objectively and subjectively by noninvasive techniques that EDTA (disodium edetate), a chelating agent will reverse the atherosclerotic process and thereby increase blood flow to the various organ systems of the body. A chelating agent is a substance which combines with heavy metals and renders them inert. The molecule then passes out of the bloodstream into the urine. Detoxification naturally occurs in the liver and the toxic waste products are removed via the lungs, kidneys, skin and feces. However, our bodies are not able to effectively eliminate the above mentioned heavy metals. EDTA up to this time has been used to successfully treat lead poisoning and has been extremely effective. EDTA is a molecular with a double tetrahedron structure and it will bind toxic heavy metals found within the cells of the body thereby helping to increase a sluggish respiratory system. This molecule is not selective in its binding properties and will leech out essential metals as well, however, these necessary trace minerals are easily replaced by taking mineral supplements such as sea salt, bone meal, or dulce.

Its strength as a healing technique lies in its effectiveness, lowered cost, and nontoxicity when compared with the grosser surgical interventions such as coronary-artery bypass surgery. Coronary-artery bypass surgery is technology's answer to technology's problems. It is a highly expensive technique costing upwards of $20,000 per operation with questionable results. It is an extremely dangerous procedure. Once again we see the folly of Western technological medicine attempting to reverse a lifetime of damage with a crude, gross intervention.

"An ounce of prevention is worth a pound of cure" is a

concept which rings deaf into the ears of the overwhelming numbers of physicians who are trained within the concepts of allopathic medicine. The result of this attitude is an overburdened, overwhelmingly expensive and ineffective health care system which is not meeting the real needs of the people. And yet the people sacrifice themselves daily to the surgeon's knife hoping for some miraculous alteration of one's health. Fortunately in California the malpractice insurance is so high regarding coronary bypass surgery that most surgeons will not risk it here anymore. An interesting paradox indeed to see economics being the force in stopping this cruel and devastating insult upon the human organism.

What is the relationship between quality, vibration, and nutrition? It has been pointed out in the *Secret Life of Plants*, that each food substance has its own vibratory rate which has been measured in angstroms. All manifestation, from people to plants to minerals, is a reflection of its vibration or energy state. Fresh, vital food still contains the essence of the life force within it. This is imparted into our bodies through the process of assimilation.

As our bodies are daily undergoing cell death and constant regeneration, it only makes sense that the substances which we put into our system will have a profound affect upon our well-being. This is why attention to quality is so important. Nonvital chemicals bring down the living essence of the food which we ingest. It is an axiom of good nutrition to try to eat fresh, vital food which has not been over-cooked as heating will break down and destroy the vital amino acids which are necessary for rebuilding body tissues.

We also need to consider the subjective aspect of what goes into eating. Proper nutrition not only involves care in selecting but concerns itself with the skill of preparation which includes the joy and creativity of cooking, how food is handled, and the manner in which it is presented and served.

All these aspects create the subjective feeling which occurs about the dining table. To be in a relaxed atmosphere enhances the food and often times what is mediocre becomes a delicious, enjoyable meal because the understanding and caring was provided.

Eating is a social act, it provides the possibility for communication and togetherness. This is the reason why food is served on religous and ceremonial occasions. The food often takes on a symbolic importance.

An example of how this works comes from my own experience. My favorite holiday is the Passover, a time of celebration, a festival of freedom. The Passover is the story of the Jewish exodus out of Egypt. During the commemoration of the Passover there is a question asked by the oldest son, "Why is this night different from all other nights?" At the time I certainly could not see behind the genius of such a question and I accepted the "stock" answers which were provided. The answer being that on this night, we, the family, behaved differently: the bread was different, the presentation and the setting of the table was different. We also were different; we all put on a different face, presented a different attitude. There was an excitement, a sense of goodwill, a desire to be kinder, to be more pleasant—a respect for the effort made by my mother to create a joyous occasion. We all consciously or subconsciously decided to forget ourselves and our problems and get into the ritual. The wine was passed, the atmosphere was mellow and we were in no rush to leave the table. Things were different because through the ritual we decided to get into the spirit of the story of the exodus.

This experience makes another point, that the theme of the exodus is the theme of freedom, not from the outside but from the inside; the realization that we all have the ability to change our conditions mentally and physically if we so choose. The point is that every day can be a celebration of life rather than on stated holidays where we allow ourselves to be more ourselves. However, the "imperatives" of the world often blind us to this very simple realization.

The next day we all reverted back to our former selves, in varying degrees, forgetting the happiness, joy and communal feeling which had been *created* the evening before. Such is life but the secret perhaps lies in the knowing that we have the choice to be positive or negative.

We can all construct and individualize our diet to our particular needs and tastes, and break through negative habits such as the excessive consumption of refined sugars. Too much sugar creates enormous metabolic upsets and it is time we moved away from our childhood addictions. The abuse of sugar intake helps to create the debilitating diseases of obesity, adult-onset diabetes mellitus and hypoglycemia, subtle nervous disorders, and general imbalance. Glucose is the energy source of the body. It is the basic substance which provides the energy to the cells needed to sustain themselves. The homeostatic mechanisms within the body are regulated to maintain a steady, balanced level of glucose circulating within the blood. Insulin is needed to move glucose across the cell walls. The adrenal steroids and glucagon are hormones which increase sugar production in time of stress and increased activity. If the body is continously bombarded with large amounts of sugar it must work harder to maintain a steady state. If the body is continually saturated from childhood with enormous amounts of sugar this affects the entire hormonal system, creating a situation where the excess must be dealt with. We become obese as this excess sugar is converted into glycogen and fat stores.

Obesity is a major medical problem in this country and reflects the lack of control and mindless addictive behavior which is fueled by an extremely ingenious and clever food and advertising industry. We are as addicted to food as we are to sex. But the pendulum is swinging back the other way as people become acutely aware that many of their medical problems can be traced *in part* to poor nutrition and eating habits. We are recognizing and demanding vital, fresh food. For example, many meats have been injected with steroids—similar substances to those found in the birth control pill. These systemic harmones are extremely powerful and exert negative influences upon the internal body. These effects are subtle but nonetheless real. Also our fruits and vegetables are sprayed with harmful chemicals which work their way into the food chain. As long as the society is quantity, not quality, oriented then there is little hope for change. However, changes will occur as we begin making intelligent choices. The law of supply and demand is as operative today as it always has been—"Ask and ye shall receive."

Our egotistic, gluttonous eating habits must change—they no longer make sense. Over-consumption creates disease, creates a profit-oriented food industry, and creates a blind neglect of a large portion of the world. The sacrifice, the changing over, can only be a positive step—we will become lighter, more mobile, freer in the sense that we will require much less than our beliefs and conditioning have taught us. We have to see past economic considerations, we have to recognize that the earth is an interdependent unity and that our physical well-being adds or detracts from the collective consciousness of our world.

High Quality Food Items

Proteins: Proteins are made of amino acids. There are twenty different types, eight are essential, that is to say they cannot be made within the body but must be ingested. Proteins are necessary for bodily repair, carry oxygen throughout the body and supply energy to the body. High quality non-meat sources of protein are peas, beans, lentils, nuts, milk, eggs, cereals, soybeans, peanuts, and wheat.

Vitamins: A balanced diet will provide a sufficient supply of vitamins. Natural sources are better than synthetic vitamins because they are artificial and processed. Something, the essence or life force of the vitamin, is lost in chemical reduplication.

Vitamin C: The anti-stress vitamin—Vitamin C has been called the anti-stress vitamin because it plays an important role in the reaction of the body to stress. Vitamin C is found in high concentrations in the pituitary gland, the adrenal cortex, and the leucocytes. In times of stress, as in the infection process, the pituitary gland secretes large quantities of Adrenocortical Stimulating Hormone which in turn produces cortisol which will affect a rise in blood leucocytes. The rise in whole blood cells is the body's response to harmful bacteria. Bacteria enter into the body when the body's resistance is lowered. Vitamin C is necessary for the production of cortisol and enzymatic reactions within the leucocytes. When the body is under stress, Vitamin C is more rapidly depleted from these vital centers, and hence it is necessary to increase one's intake of Vitamin C.

At the recent meeting of the orthomolecular medical society in San Francisco, overwhelming evidence was presented by various physicians as to the beneficial effects of vitamins in preventing and ameliorating the common cold and other infectious diseases. (Orthomolecular medicine is the treatment or prevention of illness by providing the optimum molecular environment for the mind and body. It is their concept that illness results from an imbalance within the body resulting from improper diet, exposure to toxins— heavy metals, allergens, etc.—faulty genetic inheritance, or prolonged emotional or physical stress and the resultant excesses or deficiencies which constitute the imbalance. Treatment is aimed at correcting the basic imbalance, rather than just providing symptomatic relief. Proper balance is achieved by providing the molecular environment which allows the body to heal itself. This is done by attention to basic nutrition, providing those nutrients that are found lacking or reducing those found in excess. Mineral and vitamin supplements, sometimes in large quantities are added where diet cannot fill the individual need for nutrients.)

Dr. Linus Pauling, the eminent double Nobel Prize winner, spoke to the convention reiterating the marvelous healing properties of large doses of Vitamin C in preventing the common cold. Vitamin C is found naturally in potatoes, oranges, tomatoes, cherries, and rose hips. Once again, nature provides us with what we need. Vitamin C is readily available and extremely inexpensive, and virtually non-toxic. A perfect drug.

Minerals: Minerals are necessary for many of the electrochemical reactions which are occurring continuously throughout the body. Boron, magnesium, manganese, zinc, phosphorous, calcium, copper, iodine, sulphur, and sodium bicarbonate are all necessary elements for the functioning of the body. It is imperative that we have a water supply which restores these lost elements. Excellent sources of minerals are fresh fruits and vegetables. Natural spring water, bone meal, kelp and dulce are also very rich in essential minerals.

Wheat Bran and Salads: Important because they supply the intestine with bulk that is necessary for the smooth functioning of the intestines. The high incidence in this country of carcinoma of the large intestine, diverticulitis, hemorrhoids, and chronic constipation have been related to a lack of bran and bulk in the diet.

Lower Bowel Symptomatology: The Bantu's of Africa have virtually no carcinoma of the colon, hemorrhoids, diverticular disease or hiatal hernias. Their diet includes large doses of high residue fiber (bulk). This is provided by the consumption of fruits and vegetables. Nutritionists are becoming increasingly aware of the importance of proper maintenance of the ecology of the gastrointestinal tract. Bulk is necessary to help maintain normal peristaltic activity as well as helping to create a soft, easily passable stool. The importance of bulk in the diet lies in the fact that increased intra-abdominal pressure due to excess strain while defecating, is responsible for the formation of hemorrhoids, diverticulosis and hiatal hernias. In a well-balanced diet, the normal transient time for food to pass from the mouth to the anus is approximately 12 hours. The normal peristaltic movement of the bowel moves the food forward in an orderly, rhythmic fashion— however if the autonomic nervous system is dysfunctional due to stress, anxiety, or emotional turmoil, then the transient time slows down or speeds up, depending upon the predominant emotion being elicited. This results in constipation or diarrhea.

In conjunction with abnormal transient times is the problem of the quality of food we ingest. The average American diet is high in protein, which undergoes a putrefaction process within the large bowel if it is not rapidly eliminated. This putrefaction process produces toxins and gas which poison the local bowel wall. The integrity of the local bowel wall is adversely affected, leading to localized weakening and infection secondary to what was once a friendly bacterial flora. The intrinsic peristalic movement is damaged and we have a slow, sluggish, edematous bowel wall which is no longer functioning properly. This leads to diverticulosis and diverticular disease. The stool becomes hardened and more difficult to pass as excess H_2O is removed from the bowel wall into the bloodstream. Bulk, a high residue fiber, holds back the H_2O. Not only is H_2O reabsorbed back into the bloodstream, but so are the toxins, which are the result of the on-going putrefaction process. Fortunately these toxins are detoxified by the liver, however, we should realize that a dys-

functional bowel is allowing a continual seepage of poisons
to enter into our bloodstream. This auto intoxication process
results in feelings of malaise and ill-ease, and systematically
represents a chronic poisoning of the bloodstream. All this
may be reversed by simple nutrition. A high carbohydrate
diet with emphasis on substances such as bran and psilyium
seed will reconstitute the natural ecology of the bowel wall
and decrease the incidence of carcinoma, hemorrhoids, hiatal hernias and diverticulosis. Once again an ounce of prevention is worth a pound of cure.

Food Supplements: Brewers yeast—Potent source of B-
vitamin complex.
Kelp, dulce—Trace minerals.
Wheat germ—Must be fresh; vitamin E,
vitamin B complex.
Rose hips—Vitamin C.
Lecithin—Phospholipids.
Bone meal—minerals.
Cod liver oil—Vitamins A, F, and D.
Alfalfa—Vitamins A, B-12, E, K, minerals.
Honey—Uncooked, unrefined; contains pollen,
rich in vitamins and minerals.
Yogurt—Maintains ecological balance of
intestines.

Healing Herbs

Herbs have been used throughout the centuries for healing
and relief of pain. Today's modern synthetic medicines such
as penicillin, digitalis, aspirin, morphine, quinine, are all
derived from living plants and fungi. Herbs enhance the healing process, strengthen and rejuvenate the body and purify
the blood when used in a consistent fashion. To cite just one
example which Western scientists are recognizing as a
legitimate curing substance is the chemical carbonoxolene.

This chemical is the active ingredient found in licorice root. To date, this substance has been shown to be the only substance known to cure peptic ulcer disease. It has been used successfully in Great Britain for over five years and is currently being studied at various medical schools in the United States.

As we collectively become more sensitive and aware we will learn and accept the wonderful healing abilities of herbs which have been known to the ancients both Eastern and Western for time immemorial. Also, the American Indian used herbs extensively and much of our folklore regarding the healing properties of herbs is gleaned from their wisdom.

As we begin to recognize the disastrous side effects of Western drug therapy we will return to a more natural, gentler approach to healing. So much of what is being dispensed by the pharmaceutical industry is not only ineffective but in many cases deadly in that these drugs totally upset the natural balance and rhythm of the internal processes of the body. Nature provides us with all the necessary ingredients for long life and health. We just need to recultivate our faith, re-learn scientifically the proper use of these healing elements and use them judiciously.

Healing Herbs

Alfalfa: Contains large amounts of vitamins and digestive enzymes such as *lipase*, a fat splitter; *coagulase*, coagulates milk and clots blood; *amylase*, splits starches; *protease*, digests proteins; *peroxidase*, oxidizing effect on the blood. Used as a tea it stimulates the appetite, aids in healing peptic ulcers, is a diuretic; the sprouts contain more protein than corn or wheat.

Aloe vera: This bitter tasting herb is effective for the healing of burns, skin irritations, sunburn, and insect bite.

Burdock (Arctium lappa): Considered to be an excellent

blood purifier, it cleanses and eliminates impurities from the blood; a detoxifying agent.

Chamomile (Anthemis nobilis): Excellent all-around tonic; soothes the stomach, relieves nervous tension, helps to induce sleep; soothing as a wash for sore or tired eyes.

Cascara sagrada: This is an excellent laxative; induces peristatic action of the bowels.

Cayenne (red pepper): The most powerful, natural stimulant known. Its stimulating properties increase blood flow to the tissues, therefore, it is particularly effective in rheumatism and arthritis. It is highly recommended as a means of resisting a cold.

Coltsfoot (Tussilago farfara): Excellent remedy for disturbances of the respiratory tract such as bronchitis, asthma, spasmodic coughing; soothes the mucous membranes of the lungs.

Comfrey (Symphytum officinale): Comfrey contains a substance called *allantoin*, a known cell proliferant, that can strengthen skin tissue and help heal ulcers. This herb is considered to be one of the most powerful healing herbs known. Allantoin is present in the urine of pregnant women, as well as in maternal milk, suggesting that this substance is important for the growing neonate. It has been used for asthma, the pain of gout, rheumatism and arthritis; will also increase the speed of healing of wounds, fractures, and burns. This herb is a well-recognized wonder-herb.

Dandelion (Taraxacum officinale): High in vitamin A; blood purifying and detoxifying agent, specifically for the gallbladder, urinary tract, kidneys, and spleen.

Echinalea (Echinalea augustifolia): Blood purifier; because it is a detoxifying agent it is recommended for boils, carbuncles, eczema, and acne.

Garlic (Allium sativum): This stimulant, diuretic, expectorant, and diaphoretic (sweat promoter) has been used for centuries. It is a natural antibiotic as well.

Ginseng (Panax quinquefolius): Known for its subtle rejuvenating powers, it increases the energy level of the organism. It has a stimulating effect on the central nervous system and endocrine system. Its effect is cumulative and is most effective if used consistently and in moderate doses.

Goldenseal (Hydrastis canadensis): This marvelous herb has multiple uses; it soothes and heals the mucous membranes of the body. It is useful for gastritis, cystitis, tonsilitis, sinusitis, and all catarrhal inflammations. It also is effective for ulcer diseases, be they internal or external.

Licorice (Glycyrrhiza glabra): Carbonoxolene, the active ingredient in licorice root, is effective in healing peptic ulcers.

Mistletoe (Viscum album): This herb has narcotic, antispasmodic, tranquilizing properties; effective for nervous disorders, arthritis, and headaches. The American species is a stimulant and will increase blood pressure. (The flowers and berries are poisonous, the leaves *only* are used.)

Lobelia (Lobelia inflata): The best muscle-relaxant available, it promotes an increased blood flow to the tissues thereby promoting healing by increasing oxygen to the tissues and eliminating waste. This is a true antispasmodic relaxant; because of its inherent properties as a relaxant it is particularly effective in relieving bronchiospasm which creates the symptoms of asthma. Any technique or agent which promotes relaxation of body or mind will increase the sense of well-being.

Parsley: Rich in vitamins and minerals, it cleanses internal organs and soothes the stomach.

Raspberry: Reduces pain for women in labor, increases milk supply, and helps prevent miscarriages.

Red Clover (Trifolium pratense): Detoxifying agent, blood purifier, it also has sedative properties.

Rosemary (Rosemarinus officinalis): Used in relieving nervous disorders and headaches secondary to nervous tension. Its oil serves as an excellent shampoo.

Scullcap (Scutellaria lateriflora): Excellent tranquilizer. Used in combination with other herbs to promote relaxation of mind and body.

Valerian (Valerian officinalis): Tranquilizer and antispasmodic.

Vervain (Verbena hastata): Will stimulate diaphoresis (sweating); excellent for colds, this herb has tranquilizer properties as well.

The above listing of healing and medicinal herbs is a cursory summary of the better known herbs which have been used effectively and wisely in helping to promote the healing process within the body. They are safe, gentle, and work in harmony with the body's natural processes. Nature provides man with all the necessary ingredients necessary for good health. Learning to understand the use of medicinal herbs is just another aspect of re-learning and rediscovering aspects of our essential nature. The body has fabulous healing potentials of its own and is continuously undergoing a process of death and rebirth. It is our ignorance and continuous interference with these subconscious processes which often times creates the disastrous side effects which are so common in allopathic medicine. So very often it is our mental state which creates the unfavorable healing environment in that fear, anxiety, and the expectation of failure work against the need for relaxation which is really the key to physical and mental health.

Learn to recognize the real ecological dangers that we are imposing on ourselves both internally and externally. Overcome them by judicious choices in your day-to-day process living. Learn to respect and appreciate the sanctity and incredible creation which is your living body. Learn to trust your own ideas.

Here are some guidelines which will help to effect a positive change:

1. Underconsumption—Eat balanced meals.
2. Purchase living, vital foods.
3. Learn to use herbs and spices whenever possible.
4. Be aware of your intake of trace minerals.
5. Moderately withdraw from use of synthetic drugs; try to cut down on the intake of nicotine and caffeine, find herbal substitutes.
6. Avoid processed foods containing insecticides, preservatives, artificial flavorings and colorings; avoid adulterized meat containing diethylstilbestrol and antibiotics.
7. Try to procure a clean, natural water supply.
8. Partake of fresh air and exercise.
9. Expose yourself to sunlight.
10. Learn to listen to yourself.

4

Cancer

There is probably no other pathological process which so poignantly symbolizes the collective imbalance in society today as Cancer. Cancer is a difficult subject and my intention is not that of a muckraker but of an observer who intensely feels that this dis-ease process and its treatment needs to be thoroughly reviewed and an honest recognition needs to be made based on the statistical evidence that today's medical therapies are highly ineffective, for the theoretical model upon which cancer therapy is based reflects the collective ignorance and empirical approach of orthodox medicine today. In time we will come to recognize that the cure for cancer lies in its prevention and that we are individually responsible for the creation and evolution of this disease process.

The etiology of cancer is essentially based on the premise that to stay healthy and alive we need to be expressive and creative, that all disease is basically due to insufficient energy or energy imbalances within the body. Fear, illusion and anxiety create physiological damage in themselves. This concept is simple but difficult to embrace particularly if one is thinking in terms of drugs and surgery and using Cartesian belief systems to explain reality.

Basically cancer is a systemic disease. The tumor is but a symptom of the underlying generalized process; the tumor in many cases is not the cause of death. We do not properly estimate the power of fear and anxiety in helping to create the initial disease process as well as helping to "facilitate" (in a negative fashion) the eventual death of the physical body. We must consciously realize the power of belief systems and suggestibility, particularly in a doctor-patient relationship where the patient, out of lack of self-understanding and fear, has abdicated control of the disease process. Most cancer patients place the responsibility for the establishment of the disease "outside of themselves" and this concept is reinforced by the medical profession which after 40 years of medical research cannot consistently find an etiological agent. We are becoming more aware that carcinogens, such as environmental pollutants, weaken and stress the body and thereby reduce blood flow and oxygenation to the tissues as well as disrupting cellular oxidative processes. Decreased oxygenation and impaired elimination is the initiating process of all dis-ease. We do not get cancer; it is a "creative" living process which occurs in time. It is rooted within the psyche and character development *within* the personality.

It is analogous to the concept that bacteria cause pneumonia. This is true to the extent that bacteria gain entry into the body. However, the initial causation of pneumonia is the lowering of bodily defenses, resistance or energy level. If we are weak, our resistance is low, our energy level or vibration is decreased, then we are fertile ground for the initiation of disease processes. If on the other hand, we are strong, vibrant, flowing and in balance there exists the state of health and well-being; we are much more able to resist outside influences which continuously stress and attempt to wear down our bodies' defenses. Any discipline or attitude which creates a positive, flowing existence will help to maintain a strong resistance. On the other hand, those attitudes and beliefs which create fatigue, emotional overreaction and anxiety will drain and deplete our energy stores. If man is to continue to evolve, he must realize this and know it for himself. If we understand what our lifestyles and attitudes create in ourselves, disease will be a process whereby we can see and judge the effect.

It is through this difficult learning process that often entails pain and suffering, that we come to solve the enigma of self. This requires a process of growth and change; what changes is not the world but how we see ourselves in relation to it. We may resist this change, as we have "free will," but to resist is to invite personal turmoil, to move against the currents of the universe. If we deny that love (energy) is necessary to our survival, that it nurtures and sustains us and cut ourselves off from it, then we have to accept the inevitable consequences—any one (or more) of an extraordinary range of diseases. We can be our greatest enemy, we can also be our greatest friend.

To understand the pathogenesis of this affliction we must view cancer philosophically as well as physiologically. It is our beliefs and attitudes projected onto the world which create our relative peace (ease). It is the distorted, myopic, self-conscious (egoistic) view of ourselves which creates the feelings and problems of alienation, fear and anxiety (dis-ease). As long as we perceive and feel the world as essentially hostile and take a position of opposition and non-flowingness then we are in opposition to the flow of the universe. It is man's fear and anxiety about himself and his world which creates resistance to flow and communication which ultimately creates pain, dis-ease and death. That which moves with the universe, feels its energy and is able to communicate is in harmony with all that is. For man to survive and maintain his health he must communicate, that is to give and to take, to love and accept the realization that *no*-thing exists apart from himself. It is only our separateness from ourselves that creates the illusion that we are separate from our world.

Each cell is a universe unto itself. It has a nucleus (a brain) and a cytoplasm (a body) and it exists in relation to the tissues and to the body. It fulfills its own unique function depending upon the ability of the personality to supply what it needs to support itself, and in turn it provides the necessary support, harmony, chemicals or whatever is necessary for the functioning of the whole. One cannot live without the support of the other; the body is interdependent upon the smooth functioning of the cellular units.

The body thus functions with its own Logos whereby each cell in its own inherent wisdom does exactly what is needed for the benefit of the whole also recognizing that "its" life is dependent upon the successful functioning of the whole. The cells which compose the body live in harmony and cooperation with each other supported by nutrients, oxygen, and cosmic energy.

We need to take a positive rather than negative view of creation and ourselves. We have the power to create. We are not hopeless victims to forces which reside outside ourselves. It is *only* our relative lack of understanding of ourselves which creates conflict and anxiety and imbalance. Conflict and anxiety are the basis for the pathogenesis of neoplasia.

How does a malignancy develop?

There are three concepts here which must be understood to help visualize how this process develops:

1. Movement and efficient flow are necessary to sustain life; the antithesis to flow and movement is stasis and stagnation—death.

2. Each cell lives within its own unique environment; it is dependent upon an adequate supply of oxygen and nutrients as well as an effective drainage system which is provided by the lymphatic system.

3. Each tissue is continually undergoing a continuous process of life and death—cell birth-cell death—we are in a continuous state of change, the dead cells are removed by the lymphatic system and by phagocytic action of cells called *macrophages*. Thus, for the tissues to stay alive and well the body not only must provide an adequate transport system to the cells but also an efficient system for the elimination of dead cells.

The initiating cause of cellular change or neoplasia is a result of a change in cellular oxidation.

Otto Warburg, a German Nobel prize winner in the 1930s, demonstrated that in malignant change the oxygen saturation at the tissue level was decreased. The blood gases are upset and lactic acid production is increased as a result of anaerobic cellular metabolism. In other words, the initiating cause is the relative lack of oxygen at the cellular level. If this situation is allowed to persist through time then a permanent change in the nature of the individual cells takes place; a metamorphosis occurs in response to a change in the internal milieu surrounding the affected cells. The importance of environment cannot be understated; we need to recognize that everything affects everything else.

The cells react to this changing, unfavorable hostile environment and undergo a mutation in the hopes of being able to adapt and thereby survive. The problem is that the adaptation is a maladaption which in time has disastrous consequences for the rest of the organism as the balance and harmony of the surrounding area becomes disrupted.

Thus, persistent imbalance in the oxygen and energy supply to a particular tissue will in time create a change in cellular metabolism which manifests itself as malignancy.

Remember, we are dealing with living processes. The cells "intuitively" understand that their survival is threatened and they attempt to expand as if they were searching for a new source of life.

The cancer (or crab) begins to spread out infiltrating, affecting and disturbing the normal configuration of the tissues. Some of these deranged cells seed into the blood vessels and lymphatic system and are carried to various other systems. However, their sense of harmony and balance have been destroyed; the coding and behavior of these cells are no longer under homeostatic control. They seem to have lost their sense of relationship with the surrounding healthy tissues. They no longer cohabit with their neighbors and the symbiotic relationship has been destroyed.

Other processes are occurring simultaneously. The elimination system, the lymph vessels, have been disrupted and the ordinary necrotic debris resulting from normal cellular wear and tear is not able to pass out of the system. This necrotic dead tissue also influences and affects the surrounding healthy tissue. We often see malignant cells along with areas of dead necrotic cellular debris when we examine pathological specimen of cancer tissue. This toxic debris creates fever and "helps" to poison the system thereby affecting the general metabolism of the body. This manifests in the varied presentations of cancer as symptoms such as fever, skin rashes, malaise, weight loss, pallor, decreased energy, lethargy.

It is a ghastly phenomenon to witness the body eating and destroying itself with such passion and ferocity. The body literally wastes away suffocating in its own stagnating wastes. The odor emanating from dying cancer patients often times is quite putrid, not unlike a cesspool—the person literally reeks of death.

We have stated that the initial causation of the neoplasm is decreased oxygen at the tissue level. What precipitates this?

The blood flow is intimately affected by the amount of exercise one gets as well as how aware one is of the proper control of the breathing. The autonomic nervous system is in intimate contact with the blood vessels throughout the body. In times of anxiety and prolonged stress, emotions are felt subjectively and translated into electrochemical impulses which are carried down through the spine, through the autonomic ganglia and onto the blood vessels. This interferes with the normal maintenance of a dynamic equilibrium and creates spasm and a compromised blood flow to the tissues. What we feel often in the musculature as spasm and pain may and does occur in the internal organs as well. We just do not perceive it, until we develop alarming symptoms which indicate that something is dysfunctional. Thus, if we are uptight, fearful, anxious, these emotions are reflected in the body and hinder us in many ways, not only do they create feelings of isolation and loneliness but they are draining emotions.

If we open up and express ourselves not only do our bodies become more relaxed but also the blood flow and circulation throughout the body becomes even and regulated. Breathing, inspiration and expiration, assumes a more natural flow when the higher emotions do not adversely affect the natural rhythm. To stay alive, we must be alive. We must be interested in life and therefore communicate with it.

Basically there are three concepts which I believe would help prevent cancer and could be used as therapy as well:

1. Relaxation.
2. Creativity and movement.
3. Healthy, breathing healing environment.

Relaxation

As we learn to relax, we open up ourselves to our *own* healing potentials—this permits freer flowing of our blood throughout the body as spasm is reduced.

Fear and anxiety are the opposite of relaxation. As we learn to relax we learn to see our fears and we learn to let go. It is for these reasons that the yoga philosophy, particularly Hatha Yoga, is so effective as healing modalities. Visualization techniques are extremely effective here as well as has been demonstrated by the work of Carl Simonton. The concept is essentially the same—the mind's attention is focused within and we create for ourselves scenes which are peaceful and relaxing, as the mind relaxes so does the body. We can also conceptualize ourselves being well and picture those organs which are in distress as becoming healthier. This is the potential of creative imagination, a very profound technique because we think in images. "As a man thinketh so is he."

Inspiration

One cannot underestimate the importance of *breath*—correct breathing is essential in providing us with the necessary oxygen as well as eliminating toxic by-products of metabolism. Inspiration on a subjective level leads to *creativity*. The conceptualization of a new idea creates hope, spontaneity, excitement, joy, and liveness—*if* it is real inspiration. True inspiration creates movement and action which works against the inertia of stasis and stagnation—death. In treating cancer patients, or any other dis-eased people, one must be continuously aware of the effects of hope versus despair.

The Eastern medical philosophies stress the science of breathing and are intimately aware of the necessity of movement. Movement should be controlled to avoid an anaerobic condition whereby the cells go into oxygen debt and there is an accumulation of lactic acid and other toxins which in themselves will create an unfavorable environment.

The re-creation of a healthy body takes time and the changes are subtle. We should not expect immediate results. The conflict within the cancer patient and doctor is the fear that the change must happen as soon as possible. The disease itself did not appear in one day or one week but was the result of poor living habits, a fouled environment, and negative programming. To reverse these processes takes time and understanding that the subconscious mind is responsible for the dis-ease process. Therefore, it is through the subconscious that healing will be effected through eradication of *fear* and faith in one's own healing ability.

Environment

The third ingredient necessary to reverse the cancerous process is to provide a healthy, healing environment. Hospitals as they are constructed today are wholly inadequate in providing a positive, cheerful surrounding. Most hospitals are run in an inefficient, corporate manner where time is money and the emphasis is on a short stay to help minimize severe financial strain. The problems posed by the hospital itself, a disinterested or over-worked staff for instance, compounded by anxiety over paying the bill can only exacerbate and work against the healing process. Today's hospital setting is hardly conducive to healing; those elements necessary for the healing process—fresh air, sunlight, good food, quiet environment, loving and caring, a pleasant uplifting atmosphere— are all necessary for the recovery process. Instead of building the patient's energies to effectively battle the sickness within with his own resources, we compound the situation by instilling fear, through harmful drugs and surgery. The real hope for eradicating cancer lies not in its cure but in its prevention. If different medical philosophies were employed we would see a real change in the prognosis of cancer today.

The following case history illustrates where we are now in the management of cancer, how our limited attitudes, fears and beliefs create and exacerbate a "bad" situation into a horror of overreaction and hysteria.

G. R. was on superficial appearance an outgoing, successful salesman. His wife had died seven years previous to the time he began experiencing feelings of malaise, loss of energy, change of pallor, change of posture, change of gait. Mr. R. knew that a change had occurred, he started sleeping in the afternoon, his sense of humor diminished, his sleep was interrupted by nagging dreams. G. decided to see a doctor because he just did not feel right; he was also complaining of low back pain, slight but noticeable. He went to his physician who made a diagnosis of muscular spasm and gave G. phenylbutazone, a very powerful anti-inflammatory drug used mainly in horses. The symptoms did not abate and three months later G. noticed a solid lump on his neck. Being a man with a persistent optimistic outlook, he dismissed the lump as just that. No need for alarm. Time passed, the lump remained, the depression continued. However, the situation was becoming alarming because G. was becoming progressively dyspneic (out of breath). He checked into a hospital where a massive pleural effusion (fluid in lungs) was noted and a diagnosis of lymphosarcoma was entertained and confirmed. A laparotomy was performed to determine the extent of the disease, a lymph angiogram, which was extremely painful was done to help clarify the extent of the disease. G. then underwent extensive radiotherapy along with taking cytotoxic drugs and steriods in an attempt to control the process.

He was told that the prognosis was unfavorable and that he should not expect to live more than six months, although there had been exceptions to the rule.

The "medications" created a variety of unwanted effects: His blood count fell, he became progressively anemic, his resistance to infection was interfered with. He developed pneumonia while he was being treated for his anemia. His pneumonia was successfuly treated, however, since a broad spectrum antibiotic was used, he inadvertently developed a pseudomembraneous colitis which manifested itself in a persistent bloody diarrhea. This occured because his intestinal flora was upset (the ecology of the GI tract was upset) whereby the symbiotic relationship of the bacteria changed to that of a pathogenic state. His condition was critical because of the heavy losses of fluid and potassium which further depleted his strength and energy. He recovered and was discharged from the hospital.

He continued on a regular basis with his "medication" and went back to work. His hair fell out (alopecia; side effect of cytotoxins). He became bald; he started wearing a hat and dark glasses. His self-image had crumpled and he could not face his friends; his friends had a hard time facing him as they could not deal too well with the knowledge that old, laughing, jocular, happy-go-lucky G. was dying.

His "medication" also created impotence which denied him any possibility of sexual gratification. The impotence could also be attributed to his depressed energy level as well. The steriods created pathological fractures, high blood pressure, edema in the ankles and eyes. In the course of his treatment he developed radiation sickness (persistent nausea and vomiting, destruction of oral mucosa). In time he withered away and died connected to various life support systems. It was an inglorious death, a death this man was not prepared for. All-in-all the process took place over two and half years and he received the benefit of the latest "advances" in medical technology.

The emotional and physical pain this man endured was incredible. He was partly responsible for this as he did not understand or want to understand his *dis*-ease and thereby he surrendered himself to his doctors who, operating from a limited belief system, demonstrated through the reliance upon technology a microcosm of what is wrong with medicine today. There is no doubt that his "medications," his radiation, his surgery speeded the process of death. There was no emphasis upon preparing the man for the inevitable. No real support. Today's medical model does not understand or respect the sanctity of the body or does it really want to recognize that within the body lives a personality that is experiencing fear, pain, isolation, and, in the end, terror. No one was there to really support the man in his hour of need.

He was one of many in the ward and his death was expected. It brought a collective sigh of relief because we no longer had to look at our failure and ignorance.

We acted out of ignorance and arrogance and thereby created a horror show of abuse in the rationale that what we were attempting to do was to save the man's life. An interesting paradox. And the economic considerations were astronomical—the expenses involved well over $15,000. For what?!

I spent a great deal of time with this man and we talked for hours. I found out about the real G. Here was a man in his mid 60s who as a youth was a champion athlete. He was hopelessly in love with his wife, a beautiful woman; he created an image of her after her death that no other woman could live up to. G. was sexually and emotionally tormented because on the one hand he really wanted to open up to another woman but felt it was a breach of faith.

He changed his attitude toward women that projected his deep-seated conflict. He began to see women as sex objects. Superficially he was a male chauvinist—women were objects with which to have mutual masturbation. Real contact could not and would not be made. His job was useful because he was continuously on the run. He never had time to recognize that he was running from himself and was a desperate, lonely man in search of another loving relationship.

I visited him at his home when I began to realize that cancer and most other diseases were the result of an alienation process. He was living a dangerous lie, he projected to the world the facade of a smiling extrovert, a good-time Charlie who in reality was dying inside of desperation from a lost love. He could not let that love go and saw himself as a martyr to himself. He closed himself off to real communication and thereby established a pattern which in time killed him.

We talked about death, a difficult subject to talk about

at first but a subject that needed airing. It was something he never really wanted to look at. His home reflected the desolation which he created for himself. No pictures on the wall, an old TV which he used occasionally to see a ball game. His attention span was no more than 10-15 minutes. He intimated to me before he died that he realized that he really did not want to live, however, he was afraid to die. He wanted release from his physical and emotional hell; he was caught in a vicious dilemma. Afraid to live, afraid to die.

I realized from this experience that we are responsible for our lives; we are to a large extent the creators or destroyers of our lives. I firmly believe if G. had a reason for being and found stimulation after the death of his wife, his life would not have taken such a sorry end. I also realized the unbelievable superficiality and insensitivity of mechanistic orthodox medicine. There was hardly any real human contact between staff and patient because G. was just one of many and was treated just as everybody else. A good morning, a quick survey of various blood chemistry values and a "sweet" good-bye. This is the unfortunate reality of hospital medicine today.

There is no evidence to show that the harsh methods employed created anything but further toxic processes. The rationale is to kill the cancer cells. However, this rationale has been employed for over 40 years now and the statistics are as grim as they ever have been. The radiation was radiating already dead, necrotic tissue; the scarring it created only augmented the already sluggish flow of the lymphatic system. The cytotoxic drugs further damaged and destroyed the living processes of the body and further complicated "therapy" by inducing diarrhea, baldness, anemia, susceptibility to infections. The steroids administered, while having a slight euphoric benefit, completely upset the metabolic system of this man. He was receiving these drugs in excess of 200 times the normal physiologic dosages.

(It may surprise the reader to realize that one of the most employed antimetabolic drugs used today was developed from World War I experience. Nitrogen mustards are employed extensively today on oncological services. The same substances used to poison soldiers are used today with the rationale that they can be applied to poison the tumor but not the body. A trememdous delusion indeed!)

When there is fear there is desperation, when there is ignorance there is abuse. We in the medical profession have refused to acknowledge our impotence in regards to certain disease entities. Rather than admit impotence, even when the evidence is obvious, we continue with shotgun therapies which are incredibly abusive, insensitive and economically devastating. We do not have the honesty or courage to *let it be* and provide optimal care for relief of pain and try to explore new alternatives based on the principles of *Do No Harm.*

Many cancer patients today would benefit tremendously from noninterference and supportive psychotherapy. To use a human body as a chemical experimental proving ground in the name of science is a desecration of the medical art! It should be obvious to all who study the epidemiology of cancer that the disease is not being arrested by such drastic empirical action and that the belief system which creates such inappropriate behavior must be reexamined.

Mrs. H. fits the profile of the average American housewife, 35, two children, her husband was an insurance salesman.

Mrs. H. noticed a small lump in the right outer quadrant of her left breast. She became alarmed and saw her physician who admitted her to the hospital. She was scheduled for breast biopsy with possible *radical mastectomy*—she would wake up following surgery with either a small scar or the loss of the entire breast, axillary nodes plus the underlying muscular tissue. She lost her breast. The doctors were optimistic because there was "no spread to the axilla." Breast surgery is an interesting form of exorcism. Cancer is a systemic *dis*-ease and the prognosis is *not* dependent upon what was found at surgery but upon whether or not the patient will change her attitudes and image of herself. We learn from our diseases.

This woman did not follow her prognosis. Six months later she developed bone pain and it was shown that she had developed metastatic disease. Before she died she underwent three more operations, including the removal of her ovaries, the idea being that breast cancer is somehow or other related to estrogen dependence. She was also given androgens which are male sex hormones. This created a masculinization of her body. She grew a beard. Her situation did not improve and it was decided to ablate the pituitary gland. This woman's entire hormonal system was extirpated. She underwent "chemotherapy" receiving synthetic hormones and cytotoxic drugs. Her weight steadily decreased from that of 130 pounds to a living corpse weighing 62 pounds at her death.

Is this unusual or exaggerated? I understand that the surgeons are moving away from pituitary ablation, however, what is described above is but a description of a continuous, daily occurrence in hospitals throughout the nation. This woman was never prepared for her ordeal, nor was her family, nor her children. The husband in the course of this progressive disaster developed a myocardial infarction, went financially bankrupt and had to sell their house to pay for the medical expenses.

Mrs. H. was a kind, sweet, dependable unassertive woman. She did what was expected of her, she received what she really wanted. Her sex life was next to nil—once a month—the classical story of sexual boredom in a marriage which survives only because there is a guilt obligation to keep it together for the sake of the kids. Mrs. H.'s sexual attitudes were fixed and rigid. She expressed that there was very little touching of each other's bodies, as nudity was frowned upon. There was no positive interaction between herself and her husband. She never experienced an orgasm in her life. She died acceptingly and quietly. Perhaps she did not want to upset her husband.

It was at this time that I realized that we as doctors had no real understanding of this fascinating and terrible scourge called *cancer.* Why is it I asked myself that Oriental women are not as vulnerable to the epidemic of breast cancer? I sought out a Chinese physician and spent many days and nights learning about the Taoist medical theory of energy currents within the body; how we can stimulate and maintain a healthy flow of blood, oxygen, lymph and energy to any portion of the body, through conscious consistent techniques.

Fascinating yet so simply! Perfectly in tune and derived from a philosophical base which is more highly evolved and expanded that anything I learned about or heard in medical school.

I also wondered at this time about spontaneous remissions of breast cancer. It was always known that such phenomena occurred yet it was not discussed because it did not fit into the mechanistic orthodox medical model—it was a subject which always created embarrassment to the professors who could not readily explain it within the teaching construct to which we were all exposed.

What about the women who notice lumps in their breasts and instead of developing cancerphobia *let it be*—these people never become known to us but no doubt they exist.

What effect does fear and anxiety create in the pathogenesis of breast cancer? Recently the magnitude and power of fear really hit home when I saw a woman who developed breast cancer and two months later her daughter, age 20, underwent an investigational biopsy for a lump in the breast.

The hysteria has reached epidemic proportions and a good deal of this can be attributed to Betty Ford and Happy Rockefeller's contraction of this disease. We have a situation, now in this country, of millions of women who live in constant fear of developing breast cancer; this fear being reinforced by the medical profession's advice to have multiple diagnostic tests which are equivocal.

As doctors do we really understand and empathize with the reality of what a radical mastectomy creates within the psyche of a woman? The implications and undercurrents of male surgeons performing an exorcism upon the body of a woman has many interesting psychological ramifications indeed!

The duplicity, self-righteousness and arrogance of the orthodox medical establishment is beautifully reflected in the laetril controversy.

Laetril is a substance extracted from the apricot seed and is claimed to be an effective drug in the arrest of malignancies. There is much evidence, be it subjective or empirical, that laetril has been effective in many cases. Doctors can lose their license for administering this *herb*. So it is not administered in this country. So 50,000–100,000 desperate cancer patients, unwilling to undergo the ordeal of chemotherapy and/or radiation and/or surgery seek help elsewhere. It is my belief that laetril works because the belief system is so strong that it creates a new hope and willingness to sustain oneself. There are those doctors who have attempted to explain how this herb creates a positive change at the biomolecular level. This may or may not be true—its real power lies in the power of suggestion along with its innocuousness. It does not create side effects. It does not create further stress upon the internal milieu of the body. It is not adding insult to injury. It is an incredibly powerful placebo which triggers creative action and *hope* in the patient. His or her recovery is really dependent upon the sustaining of a consistent acceptance of life and the desire to live. The AMA calls this *quackery* and will in no uncertain terms ostracize a physician who basically is trying to spare the patient the horrible ordeal of hospitalization. It is this hypocrisy and flagrant misuse of power which drives so many sensitive, aware, psychologically oriented physicians to distraction. The one thing we know about laetril is that it is harmless when administered in physiological dosages.

At this point I would like to list the undesirable side effects possible from the use of some "chemotherapeutic" agents in the treatment of cancer.

Steroids

Fluid and Electrolyte Disturbances: Sodium retention; fluid retention; congestive heart failure in susceptible patients; potassium loss; hypokalemic alkalosis; hypertension.

Musculoskeletal: Muscle weakness; loss of muscle mass; osteoporosis; vertebral compression fractures; aseptic necrosis of femoral and humeral heads; pathologic fracture of long bones.

Gastrointestinal: Peptic ulcer with possible subsequent perforation and hemorrhage; pancreatitis; abdominal distention; ulcerative esophagitis.

Dermatologic: Impaired wound healing; thin fragile skin; petechiae and ecchymoses; erythema; increased sweating; burning or tingling, especially in the perineal area (after intravenous injection); allergic dermatitis; urticaria; angioneurotic edema.

Neurologic: Convulsions; intracranial pressure with papilledema usually after treatment; vertigo; headache.

Endocrine: Menstrual irregularities; development of Cushingoid state; suppression of growth in children; secondary adrenocortical and pituitary unresponsiveness, particularly in times of stress as in trauma, surgery, or illness; decreased carbohydrate tolerance; manifestations of latent diabetes mellitus; increased requirements for insulin or oral hypoglycemic agents in diabetes.

Ophthalmic: Posterior subcapsular cataracts; increased intraocular pressure; glaucoma; exophthalmos.

Metabolic: Negative nitrogen balance due to protein catabolism.

Others: Anaphylactoid or hypersensitivity reactions; thromboembolism, weight gain, increased appetite, nausea, malaise, psychological and/or physiological dependency.

Side Effects of Steroids: Rare instances of blindness. Hyperpigmentation or hypopigmentation; subcutaneous and cutaneous atrophy; sterile abcess; charcot-like arthropathy.

The incidence of unwanted effects depends on dosage and duration of therapy but may occur in as many as 50 percent of cases.

Cytotoxic drugs

These drugs are cellular poisons. They destroy the cancer cells as well as destroying proliferating healthy tissues. This manifests as anemia, leucopenia, thrombocytopenia (decreased platelets which lead to bleeding disorders), exfoliation of intestinal mucosa, bloody diarrhea, loss of hair, impotence.

Statistics over the last 20 years have shown conclusively that

CANCER SURVIVAL*

Five Years after Diagnosis

	Stomach	Colon	Rectum	Lung and Bronchus	Kidney	Bladder	Melanoma of Skin
Women:							
1950-59	13%	46%	42%	11%	36%	53%	60%
1960-69	14%	46%	41%	12%	38%	55%	73%
Men:							
1950-59	12%	42%	38%	7%	32%	55%	51%
1960-69	10%	42%	37%	8%	36%	56%	55%

	Breast	Cervix Uteri	Corpus Uteri	Prostate
Women:	60%			
1950-59	60%	59%	71%	
1960-69	63%	57%	72%	
Men:				47%
1950-59				47%
1960-69				52%

*Percentages are based on a relative survival rate of the observed surviving divided by the proportion expected to survive in the general population based on mortality rates current during the period; study includes only white men and white women. Based on statistics from statistics from the National Cancer Institute as computed by the Statistical Bureau of the Metropolitan Life Insurance Company.

this modality does not significantly affect the over-all life span or prognosis of the patient. These drugs cannot be justified anymore. The statistics speak for themselves, yet new studies with "new drugs" which are but variations of the original drugs, go on. Human beings are still being used in protocols to help "prove" the worthwhileness of this or that modality. The quality of life, the cost and psychological damage, the pain, the despair are factors which are known yet are not primary considerations—if considered at all.

The extreme irony of the situation regarding cancer therapy is the irrational attacks of the so-called experts against any of their colleagues who dare try a different, less lethal, approach to cancer control; there is ample evidence, particularly in Europe, that cancer can be eradicated through diet, exercise and induced fevers. Oriental medicine which is integrative would never go to the extreme that we do. The underlying cause for our overreaction is deeply imbued with cultural conditioning which will not accept, or at least has a difficult time accepting, death. Our culture also refuses to recognize that man must exist with nature and cannot dominate it—this reflects in our approach to medicine.

What is the purpose of attempting to "save" a patient's life when the quality of life is destroyed? If we really looked at it clearly we would see the irrationality of it. We explored the intimate, sensitive relationships of the glandular system of the body and discovered that if the glandular system is balanced and intact then we enjoy health. The insulting of the body chemistry with massive unphysiological doses of extraordinarily toxic, powerful "drugs" has no rationale in science or any other philosophy. What we are witnessing is a desperate struggle to conquer something which we fear immensely because we do not understand it. Fear creates irrationality and desperation. The feelings of frustration and despair are known to doctors who manage cancer patients. These are not evil, malicious people but they are misguided

—always hoping that they will cure someone, never realizing or admitting that should this happen—and it does—the testimony goes to the strength and determination of the patient. Not only has the patient overcome the inherent problem which manifests as cancer, he has also overcome the negative unconscious feelings of his doctors and friends who abide by a belief which is persistently unoptimistic. And it is a supreme tribute to the incredible healing potentials of the body that it can withstand and resist a massive assault of drugs or radiation or surgery or combinations of all three in an atmosphere which is hardly conducive to ultimate recovery.

Most doctors see themselves as clinicians as opposed to healers, but all we can really do is to provide the setting for healing to take place as well as instill that subjective, non-quantifiable aspect called faith. But before we can instill this into another human being we must have faith within ourselves and believe in the type of medicine which we practice. This lack of faith, both within the medical community and with the "consumers" is the element which has created the malpractice fiasco.

Machines, advanced technology, synthetic drugs are limited. They have their place, in the background, not in the foreground. We in the healing profession have succumbed to the illusion of glamour and have engaged in a form of sophisticated cookbook medicine unable to see past the world of appearances. We need to reform medicine as a creative art. We must recognize that we are collectively responsible for the enormous pathology and disease which we see in this country. Medicine cannot be successful if it continues to operate totally from an economic base, our sense of humanity must have top priority.

The cancer "industry" is presently spending $35 billion a year in detection, research and treatment. As long as we view this dis-ease as something which must be fought and defeated we will continue to allow this enigma to strike down millions of Americans daily, with no real hope of cure because, like all internal dis-eases, it is an *idea* which if continually reinforced through suggestion manifests itself.

Innovation is desperately needed in medicine today; we need courage. The education of the people and of the doctors needs to undergo a drastic change. Medical school should not be a torture chamber where one is inculcated with theoretical data which are irrelevant in the light and reality of day-to-day medical practice. The human touch needs to be reestablished!

Communication and contact—caring—are essential. These are the real opiates and these are the factors which really influence the course and nature of illness. To ignore these truths is to continue the delusion which will perpetuate a medical system devoid of credibility, reeking in its own bureaucracy and experiencing failures which benefit no one. What we are seeing is the power of the collective ego and its attendant folly. It's encouraging to see some people attempting to establish control over their lives. We have been misled and at the same time we have misled ourselves. We have seen the enemy and the enemy is US. The enemy is ignorance and the lack of faith in one's self; we have the ability and resources not only to heal ourselves but to know what is necessary for a healthier, more satisfying life. Through the process of evolution and self-understanding which often entails suffering we will learn that health and well-being are the essential and natural states of man. It is within this deeper understanding that freedom lies. For those who do not yet understand these concepts or ideas, all they have to know and to remember is to ask for help.

5

Anxiety — Depression

Anxiety

Anxiety is a subjective state of emotional stress and ill-ease
that is reflected in the body by feelings of tightness and tension which tend to be of a prolonged nature. Anxiety is a prolonged state of fear due to subconscious processes which cannot be consciously understood by the person who is feeling it.
The higher energy or higher self is not consciously being experienced and we view life as an opposition of forces which
create pain and suffering. Anxiety in time creates numerous
disease entities and it is for this reason that we must learn to
relax our bodies and minds to allow healing energies to flow
through us. Not knowing ourselves creates energy imbalances and blocks within us. This manifests as muscular
tension, hypertension, heart disease, ulcers, and virtually
every other *dis*-ease prone to man. Thus the formulae of anxiety, tension, energy blocks, and *dis*-ease are immutable. Our
bodies are the key to our conscious growth. The more we
learn to relax and to let go, the greater the energy flow, the

greater our own personal ease, the greater the feeling of well-being residing within. The road to inner peace, health and happiness lies in the ability to express oneself and to be able to relax, and flow with life. Because of limited and distorted value systems and priorities, which are essentially materialistic in nature, we only see and react to a limited view of reality and this myopic vision creates feelings of competition, struggle, inner and outer turmoil, confrontation and *dis*-ease. We are constantly in a hurry both in a physical sense and in our mental processes. We are going nowhere fast. The old adage of slow down and live is as valid today as it was 100 years ago.

Anxiety is the result of worry and fear, usually over matters which are buried in the past or possibilities in the future. Tension and stress are created through overreaction and a feeling of not being faithful to your own expectations of yourself. Our emotional well-being is dependent upon our ability to satisfy our aspirations, to understand the reality of our true spiritual nature and to recognize the spiritual nature of whomever comes into our environment. There is nothing more devastating than the emotions of loneliness and alienation. It is imperative to live a life of relative balance, to know you are never out of the universe, that you are an intimate part of it. The experience of being one with the universe is self-revealing. However, it is only self-revealing while one is experiencing it. It is a subjective, powerful, experience to realize that you are surrounded by creation and live in relation with all that is. It is how we live within our experience that creates our personal reality. It is the nature of personal reality which we quantitate and call health.

It is our conditioning and beliefs which reflect as *attitude*, which moves us through our experience. As long as we see life in terms of duality and separation, as us versus them, we will experience fear and anxiety. Fear and anxiety are the results of not knowing who we are and thereby not knowing

who "they" are. This blindness and confusion creates a disharmony associated with negative belief systems. We are as
we think we are, we are as we do.

The nature of the universe is to move toward dynamic
equilibrium. This process of achieving balance requires
recognition that you are out-of-balance, that you are experiencing pain, and you have the desire to seek balance, to reed-
ucate and redirect your life.

It is interesting to note that one-fourth of all adults are
"supposedly" suffering from hypertension. It is also interesting to note that medical researchers are still not able to
explain the cause of this national "calamity." The cause lies
within ourselves and its solution does too.

The Causation of Primary Hypertension

Before we can successfully treat a disease or a condition we
must be aware of the causation of the problem. In orthodox
medicine the cause of hypertension is said to be "unknown."
The term *idiopathic* or *essential hypertension* is hypertension
without apparent cause. The word *hypertension* itself gives
its probable causation—increased tension or stress.

As we become more aware of the relationship between
the psyche and the soma we may postulate that the real problem with hypertensives is their maladjustment to the strains
and stresses of life. There is an intimate relationship between
the higher emotions and their effects upon the physiology and
biochemistry of the body. Man is a psychophysiological
organism who elaborates both hormonal and electrochemical impulses in a rhythymic, biofeedback manner.

The key to understanding and treating hypertension
resides in teaching the individual the ability to relax and to
relate to the world in such a manner that his life's experience
brings meaning and harmony to himself rather than stress,
fear, and anxiety.

The relationship between the higher emotions and the physiological processes occurring moment to moment within the body is the basis of psychosomatic medicine. The philosophy which is becoming more and more accepted in medical circles today recognizes the immediate relationship between projected attitudes and behavior as intimately affecting bodily and mental health. The relationship between the higher centers of man and the autonomic nervous system, mediated through the parasympathetic and sympathetic nervous system, is one of immediate and direct connection. For example, the blood pressure's homeostatic mechanisms within man are controlled in the medulla oblongata found in the brain stem. The control of blood pressure, respiration and heart rate is controlled automatically below the level of our conscious awareness. That is to say, we do not have to think about our hearts beating, our lungs respiring, and our blood pressure maintaining itself. It may be said that this mechanism is subconscious; it is going on but we are not aware of it. The body when it is relaxed and functioning normally and is not subjected to undo stress will maintain itself in a dynamic equilibrium.

When we examine the nervous system we must realize it is the product of millions of years of evolution, and by this process we have developed a hierarchy of cascading levels of control. Our higher emotions of how we feel about ourselves and our world has a direct influence upon the vital centers which control the basic neurophysiologic centers of our body. These feelings or emotions are transmitted to the pituitary gland and to the autonomic nervous system as hormonal and electrochemical impulses. Hypertension is the result of increased peripheral resistance in the arterioles of the abdominal viscera particularly those affecting the kidneys.

In times of stress we respond physiologically to the appropriate stimuli. The body will elaborate those hormones

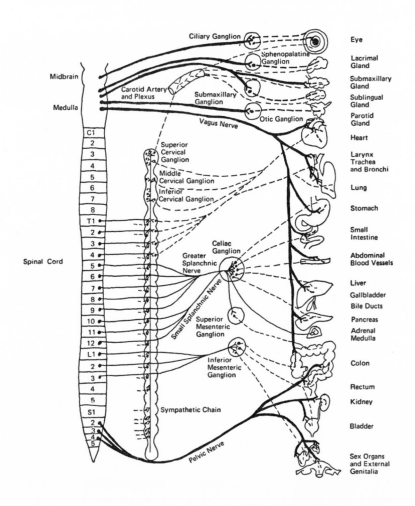

Diagram of the Efferent Autonomic pathways. Pregarglionic neurons are shown as solid lines, Postgarglionic neurons as dotted lines. The heavy lines are Parasympathetic fibers, the light lines are sympathetic.

which are necessary to increase oxygen to the tissues, increase the blood glucose level, and raise the blood pressure so that there is greater energy available for action. However, if an individual is in a state of chronic stress, worry, turmoil, or fear he will maintain a raised blood pressure and an irregular respiration. This problem is an inappropriate response to his experience. The hypertension reflects a chronic persistent neurochemical imbalance, which manifests itself clinically as an elevated blood pressure. These people tend to exhibit reactory behavior patterns which are based upon regative thinking processes. Energy follows thought and if our thoughts are predominantly angry, fearful, or worrisome they will create an over-discharge of the sympathetic nervous system which creates arteriolar spasm and hypoxia. This over-stimulation of the sympathetic nervous system will create such phenomena as hypertension, tachycardia, sweating, and general gastrointestinal tract disturbances.

It is easy to see the rationale for modern drug therapy for hypertension and also its limited effect due to all the undesirable side effects. These drugs work on the effect as opposed to the cause; they work on the autonomic ganglions and block the nervous discharge thereby relieving spasm, hypoxia, and resultant hyperexcited feedback loops which maintain the elevated blood pressure. However, these drugs do not work selectively and while they do create a lowered blood pressure or sedation they also interfere with the other normal homeostatic mechanisms of the autonomic nervous systems. For example, rauwolfia drugs create nasal stuffiness, sodium retention, gastric hyperacidity, and often severe depression; hydralazine may cause headaches and palpitations with tachycardia. Acute hypotensive reactions are manifested by weakness, nausea, vomiting, and faintness; acute or progressive renal failure due to decreased renal blood flow or filtration pressure. Vascular thromboses and renal failure are hazards in older patients who suffer severe

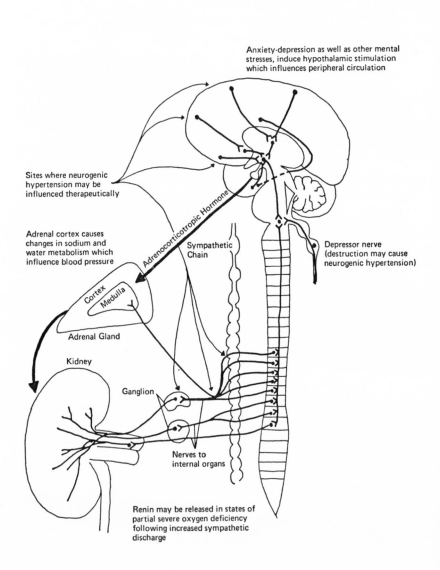

Anxiety-depression as well as other mental stresses, induce hypothalamic stimulation which influences peripheral circulation

Sites where neurogenic hypertension may be influenced therapeutically

Adrenal cortex causes changes in sodium and water metabolism which influence blood pressure

Adrenocorticotropic Hormone

Sympathetic Chain

Depressor nerve (destruction may cause neurogenic hypertension)

Cortex

Medulla

Adrenal Gland

Kidney

Ganglion

Nerves to internal organs

Renin may be released in states of partial severe oxygen deficiency following increased sympathetic discharge

Pathways in Neurongenic and Humoral Hypertension

and abrupt falls of blood pressure. Parasympatholytic effects due to parasympathetic blocking by the ganglionic blocking agents will cause blurring of vision, constipation, dryness of the mouth, and impotence.

Up to this point we have concentrated on the autonomic nervous system and its relationship to the various organs and blood vessels of the body. However, in studying the relationship between the cerebral cortex, the hypothalamus, the pituitary gland and the adrenal cortex, one may discover how a dysfunctioning of this feedback system can create a disequilibrium of the body's chemistry and thereby lead to dis- ease.

The hormones derived from the adrenal cortex are steroids. The structure, growth and secretory activity of the adrenal cortex are regulated entirely by the anterior pituitary gland which secretes a substance called *adrenocorticotropic hormone* (ACTH). This causes the release into the blood stream of cortisone or cortisol. The production of ACTH is inhibited by the release of cortisol or cortisone into the bloodstream. If there is a fall in the cortisol level, ACTH secretion commences through a so-called "servomechanism" and, thereby, raises the cortisol level again, which turns off ACTH. This continuous feedback inhibition of ACTH by cortisol may be interrupted at any time by an overriding mechanism, such as stress. Stressful stimuli reaching the cerebral cortex release the inhibition of the reticular formation or of the limbic system upon the hypothalamus. Large neurons then secrete corticotropin-releasing factor (CRF). The CRF travels down the portal circulation of the pituitary stalk to the anterior pituitary, releasing ACTH, which activates the adrenal cortex. The greater the stress, the more ACTH is secreted, and hence the more cortisone is produced. These hormones are called *glucocorticoids*. These are catabolic hormones and have a profound effect upon the proper functioning of the body. An imbalance of these hormones is directly responsible for various disease states. They lead to diversion of amino acids from muscle to the liver for deamination. Muscle wasting with weakness results. Decreased protein synthesis and increased resorption of bone matrix occur.

Amino acids that are blocked from entry into muscle go to the liver, where they are deaminated, the carbon skeletons forming carbohydrate (notably glycogen) and fat. This increased gluconeogenesis raises the blood glucose which is immediately reduced by increased excretion of insulin from the beta cells of the pancreas. However, these will eventually become exhausted in people with poor insulinogenic reserve, leading to diabetes. Excess glucocorticoids lead to a rise in serum lipids and cholesterol. This is highly significant in that it is well-recognized that increased lipids and cholesterol are intimately related to atherosclerotic heart disease. This is a metabolic problem arising not so much from dietary indiscretion but from chemical imbalances created by undue stress upon the normal physiological and biofeedback systems of the body.

"The well-developed atherosclerotic plaque is a result of the interplay of inflammatory and reparative processes. Electron microscopy has shown that these plaques are often accompanied by an abnormal intracellular storage of lipids, particularly cholesterol esters, fatty acids and lipoprotein complexes. These findings have strengthened the thesis that lipid infiltration from the bloodstream may be a significant factor in the growth of the atheromatous plaque" (CIBA Collection, *The Heart*).

Excess steriods increase gastric acidity, with a greater secretion of hydrochloric acid and pepsin and a thinning of mucus in the stomach, aggravating ulcers already present or predisposing to ulcer formation.

Changes in calcium metabolism lead to a marked increase in renal excretion of calcium, decreased absorption of it in the intestines by counteracting vitamin D, and bone effects as mentioned above. Together with a catabolic attack on bone matrix, a creeping osteoporosis (weakening and softening of the bones) is induced when excess cortisol is present.

Retention of sodium at the renal tubular level occurs. Exchanging with the reabsorbed sodium at the tubular level, potassium and hydrogen are secreted, so that cortisol excess leads to potassium depletion, weakness and alkalosis.

Cortisol diverts amino acid from lymphoid tissue as well, leading to marked reduction in size and to actual lysis of the nodes. This is accompanied by an initial release of antibodies stored in lymph nodes but, eventually, by a marked decrease in overall antibody production, which, together with breakdown of inter- and intracellular barriers to the diffusion of particles, raises susceptability to viral and bacterial infections.

An overall increase in neural excitability, with a lowered threshold for epileptic seizures, is found on the one hand, marked excitability and sleeplessness on the other.

The blood picture is markedly affected by cortisol giving rise to lymphocytopenia (decreased lymphocyts) and marked eosinopenia (decreased eosinophils) in the fact of significant neutrophilia (increased neutrophils). This explains the anti-inflammatory action of cortisol. The cellular response to a noxious or infectious agent is reduced by decreasing the accumulation first to neutrophils and second of lymphocytes, and finally by inducing delayed fibroplasia. Thus, the exudative inflammatory response is abolished. In the same manner, cortisol is anti-allergic and both a decrease in the formation of histamine and histamine-like substances by the affected cells and some surface protection of cells that would normally react to an antigen-antibody complex are involved. These actions of glucocorticoids form the basis of their widespread clinical use. As inflammatory and allergic responses are decreased, eventual fibrosis is minimized and subsequent

degeneration reduced. Thus, cortisol abolishes manifestations of disease without directly antagonizing the causative
agent.

Physiologists have been concerned for some time with
the visceral and other physical manifestations of emotional
states, but until recently the emotions themselves were almost
exclusively in the province of the psychologists. The dis-
covery that the hypothalamus and the limbic system of the
brain are intimately concerned not only with emotional expression but with the genesis of emotions has now brought
the fields of physiology and psychology closer together. What
we think and what we think about creates our feeling states.
A person in love thinks differently than a person who is
angry, fearful or lonely.

Our problem is really one of gaining control of our own
mind. As children we are taught and educated as to the
nature of reality. We become conditioned to see and perceive
the world in a certain way. The truth of the matter is that
most people at this point in evolution perceive their life and
their experience dualistically and hence negatively. These
negative thought forms or attitudes reflect themselves not only in behavior but in physiological states. Remember, the
vital centers which subconsciously control the entire physiology of the body are under the direct control of the self-conscious or higher centers of the brain. Our conscious thoughts
directly impress themselves upon our subconscious, creating
various responses which are felt within the body. Our minds
can make us sick but they can also make us healthy.
"Healthy mind, healthy body."

Our problem is one of reconditioning and relearning
faulty habit patterns based on continuous reactionary behavior. As we learn to gain control of ourselves and our emotions
we become more relaxed, peaceful, and happier, from this we
experience greater degrees of freedom. We may come to
realize ourselves as expanding beings who already have

enough and realize that true peace, happiness and freedom is a state of mind, an internal affair based upon the realization that our true nature is sublime and infinite. The clearing and changing of our consciousness and thereby our energy state is basically a re-educational process.

Hypnosis and self-hypnosis are modalities or techniques which allow us to consciously reprogram our subconscious so that these two aspects, self-conscious and subconscious, coexist in harmony. The process of self-hypnosis and autosuggestion allows an individual to learn to relax himself at will thereby gaining control over himself.

Eastern yogis are adept in self-hypnosis. The yoga philosophy is a system of autosuggestions whereby through practice and continuous reinforcement the individual gains conscious control of his subconscious and thereby learns to gain control over his own body. The subconsious controls the autonomic nervous system as well as the pituitary gland. It is totally responsible for the health and well-being of the body. Subconsciousness is always amenable to control by suggestion. Hypnosis is the art whereby the rational, intellectual mind is suspended and access is gained directly into the subconscious. Thus, under hypnosis a person who is generally nervous, upset or worried will experience profound relaxation and relief. This occurs because the subconscious is responding to suggestions from the doctor or operator to relax.

To be healthy and happy it is imperative that we learn how to relax at will. Learning to hypnotize yourself is an easily learned art, however, it must be taught by a competent teacher because the art lies in the language. The formulations of the suggestions are critical; if they are positive and direct then the desired results will be realized. Negative suggestions create negative happenings; positive suggestions create positive happenings.

An analogy which I find helpful to show how hypnosis works is that of a plant in a pot. The subconscious represents the soil. You place the seed (the idea) into the soil, water it occasionally and lo and behold, a flower grows. All very mysterious, all happening beneath the level of conscious awareness. If the idea or seed is negative, weeds grow instead of flowers. What is required of us is to know what it is that we want. The subconscious or soil will elaborate what it is that we desire. It is always amenable to suggestion, it is always receptive to self-consciousness. We have the innate power to change our personal circumstances.

Disease may be reversed by learning the art of relaxation which may be achieved through a process of self-hypnosis. The subconscious is not only receptive to self-conscious impulses but is also receptive to the self or the superconscious. Through relaxation and faith in self we may witness the reverse of many so-called terminal disease processes. This relationship explains the phenomenon of faith healing and telepathic communication as well as the power of blessings and prayer.

If we understand that we are part of one mind and share a collective subconscious then we may apprehend the power that lies within us. If we realize that energy follows thought and words are symbols which convey ideas, then we may be able to imagine ourselves as healthy and happy. This concept of an active imagination expressed through positive, courageous words, reinforced periodically, is the basis of hypnosis. Because the hypnotic technique talks directly to the subconscious we may bring about harmony within the neuro-edocrine system. Through a process of consistent reinforcement we will be able to change negative subconscious thinking patterns into positive thought forms and thereby begin to experience ever greater degrees of peace and happiness. The responsibility however lies within the individual to begin to recognize what it is he wants to change and then to formulate the proper suggestions to bring about the desired aims. We all have access to unlimited energy; we all have the ability to heal ourselves or allow ourselves to activate those aspects of subconsciousness to speed up the healing process.

Once we begin to realize and appreciate that the universal mind or life is a life always working toward our own liberation then we may realize that life is a blessing, an adventure in consciousness and self-understanding. Those same laws which appear to be working against us as one experiences the pain, may be used in a positive way and thereby reverse negative circumstances. It is only the illusion of separateness and ignorance which creates misunderstanding and pain. We can begin to build, strive, and create ourselves over in a fruitful, positive way. It is only our doubts, our over-intellectualization of experience which hide the truly magnificent nature of our true selves and this incredible universe in which we find ourselves.

Depression

Depression is a relative term and is a reflection of our energy state. When we say that we are depressed we are expressing a negative viewpoint. The associated characteristics of depression are those of boredom, listlessness, futility, lack of desire, a sense of inertia, lack of spontaneity, lack of creativity, loss of humor; the sleep rhythm is often disturbed, the appetite is generally poor, work performance declines, decline in physical activity, there is a disinterest in social interaction, one may become morbid and suicidal; if this state persists it may precipitate a psychotic break with vivid "negative" hallucinations.

We call such an experience a mental disease. The person who experiences these negative spaces develops a slow gait, the facial color changes, the head is usually bent downwards, the eyes are dull and glazed—it is obvious to all that this person has lost touch with his environment and with himself; he is cut off from his own energy source and from the possible energy sources of others. There is an intuitive knowingness among people that depressed individuals are not particularly pleasant to be around and that they exert a toxic influence around those with whom they interact. These unfortunate people are toxic, draw energy from others, and therefore have a negative influence on their environment. It is for this reason that health workers or family who associate with depressed individuals must be strong and positive within themselves. The attitude of acceptance, the recognition that this is a process that in time will be corrected will help create an equilibrium and positively influence the person in need of assistance.

We should be aware that a depressed person has created this space for himself and has the power to *un*-create it. To yell, scream, beseech, threaten or attack such an individual will only reaffirm the state in which he is struggling to leave. The cause of the depressive episode resides within the psyche of the human being and it is a reflection of an imbalance and should motivate him to explore and examine the processes creating these mood shifts. Time is the great healer and in time the feelings will change. What precipitates the change is usually known only to the experiencer and guessed at by the doctor, however, the change from one mood to another is always governed by a change in the level of energy.

It is a dramatic, exciting event to witness a person who 24 hours before was living in a personal hell—contemplating many inglorious exits, cursing life, seeing no hope whatsoever, seeing life as a cruel hoax played upon him by an unmerciful God—to change to a laughing, smiling, partially ashamed, energetic, purposeful, excited human being. The gait, attitude, facial expressions, sexual interest, sleep patterns, appetite, all change in unison.

The body, the physical reality, the biorhythm which it is subject to is real. However, it reflects tendencies and possibilities, not irrevocable happenings. Man has free will, the spirit resides beyond the limitations of time and physical reality. Through a process of knowing oneself we can see and know our high times and our low times, and thereby adjust to them. We recognize the forces which create these changes and by employing various personal techniques we modify and flow with these forces which exude such a profound effect upon the course of our lives.

It is interesting to note here that medical science is just beginning to recognize the possibility that astrology may be a valid art, that our moods (and more) may be influenced by the sun, moon, planets, and stars. This conflict brings to light a clinical situation in which a patient was trying to explain why her behavior was so bizarre. Her explanation was highly detailed with astrological terminology—"her moon was conjuncted with such and such a planet which is transiting in such a way that it creates a particular effect." The psychiatrist wanted to explain her behavior in terms of analytic concepts so that it would make sense to him. She persisted stating that both systems are just methodologies of explaining phenomena. The language of the "patient" was foreign to the doctor just as the doctor's "explanation" of what was going on was foreign to her. He read his books, she read her books; both insisted that each was valid; both are. Both systems are an attempt to gain self-understanding and being systems of thought and doctrine they are therefore limited. Words and absoloute belief systems create limitations. The story has a nice sequel to it—the patient realized that she was unable to control those forces within herself and felt that she was a danger to herself. She asked for help. The psychiatrist was "opened" enough to acknowledge that astrology might have some credibility. He did not use it as further proof of her bizarre behavior.

A compromise was made. She was placed on a tricyclic

antidepressant and they agreed that in time she should improve. She went along with the game plan because she
recognized her distress and the ridiculousness of her having
to prove that astrology was a proven system. She was going
through a difficult time and anticipated that things would be
easing up by the end of the month when her planets would be
more favorably situated. Three weeks later she was much improved, a totally different personality. The psychiatrist
credited the amtryptyline; the patient, thankful and happy,
credited the natural progression of things, rooted in a firm
belief "that all things must pass." As a neutral observer to
this interesting interaction, I credited the "cure" to the belief
inherent in the patient that she would get better, along with
the doctor's belief that the medication would help her. The
situation would have been different and less smooth had the
patient not accepted the medication because she would have
denied or resisted the reason she came for help. What is potentially dangerous here however is the misinterpretation of
why she got better. She got better because she wanted to and
because she got support for her belief system. To tell her
overtly or covertly that she is deluded and her beliefs regarding astrology are wrong would have undermined the entire
therapy.

Confrontation between modern orthodox medical
models and the occult art of astrology lead me to recognize
the profound reality of cycles and periodicity. We in the
health profession need to detach ourselves from the concept
that we are effecting the cure. A cure is never permanent,
and its occurrence cannot be ascribed to a pill or drug. It's
just not that simple.

People who find themselves in the midst of severe pain,
mental anguish, disharmony, need support, guidance and
compassion—what they do not need is electroconvulsive
therapy, coercion, massive drug therapy, a label. Any one of
us can and has manifested very unpleasant behavioral disorders. Most of us have been able to keep our private insani-

ties to ourselves and not expose these aspects to "others." The
sooner we recognize and learn to accommodate abnormal
behavior as part and parcel of the life experience the closer
we will move toward true freedom of expression.

Depression is emotional pain. Depression is a product of ego
projection mechanisms. It is a process caused by emotionally
backed desires, demands or addictions which are not being
met by outside circumstances. It can be a means of growth if
we can understand the pain as an indication of a conditioning or program being filtered through us, causing a particular reaction. Reaction is the key and one needs only to
analyze the situation which precipitates this change.

We should remember that depression is basically the result of
blocked energy flow. The pain, and it can be excruciating, is
psychophysical in that we consciously or unconsciously
block our feelings. (*Feelings* are emotive energy forms expressed in various modes be they words, movement, art or
whatever.) It is our inability or desire not to communicate,
not to express ourselves, which creates the tensions and anxieties. To live we must communicate—communication is the
key to our existenace. It is the energy flow which we share
with each other. It is what stimulates us. It is what excites us.
It is what makes the daily drama of our lives what it is. It is
our inhibitions, which are a product of conditioning with
resultant feedback loops based on programmed reactive
behavior, which impede this energy flow.
    It is our fear and lack of self-esteem and feelings of un-
worthiness that often prevents us from speaking or expressing
what we truly feel. We fear censure or ridicule not knowing
often that what we say is just as relevant, just as important,
as any other human being with whom we share time and
space—the fact that our experience may be different than someone else's does not render it unimportant or irrelevant.
    No other person can be our own best authority. An at-

titude of subservience creates a sense of inferiority and is an abnegation of the awareness that we are sentinent beings, expressions of energy in a particular form. Our bodies are but symbols with which we communicate. It is only a distorted, limited view of beauty which creates so much of our negative reaction to all that crosses our path. It is these encounters which allow an opportunity to grow and expand our awareness, recognizing the uniqueness of every man, woman and child.

Depression can be seen as a withdrawal from life, a fear of living, a feeling of uselessness and purposelessness, a denial of who we really are. Often, it is a long, arduous journey but once we recognize our lives as a process we can better face the vicissitudes and challenges which confront us day-to-day.

We have to apply a great deal of energy to remain miserable and depressed because our nature is to advance and progress. We are in an ever-moving universe and to resist its inherent, expansive nature is to try to resist forces which are much greater than any individual. Once we become consciously aware that we have the power to correct or change any mood or emotion through will and directed action then we are in a position of self-responsibility. We can no longer blame others for our emotional status; our awareness makes it clear that our reactions have created our own here-and-now feelings.

We can be our own worst enemy. Genuine help is often violently rejected in rages of self-pity and self-contempt. "Why help me?—I am just a no good son-of-a-bitch!" Because we feel so unloving we cannot accept genuine love or help from another who may see the situation objectively and offer assistance. This is a crucial point in therapy; a person must be open or ask for help when he is experiencing pain. Fortunately, in time, the situation becomes so intolerable that one moves out of it, however, our moods and emotions have effects upon other people who may react in a negative fashion. This can destroy a family, sabotage work relations, destroy a love relationship.

As you allow your emotional reactions to rule you will see the world as a reinforcing reality. You will see the world as confused, unhappy, miserable, without meaning, even though you are fully unaware that it is your perception which creates the reality. As the negative attitudes and withdrawal pass away, along with the fear, then you may perceive the world full of communicating human beings, struggling with basically the same problems, attempting to solve their own particular situation in their owner manner.

We all have scars from influences which were less than ideal be they parents, brothers, educators, the mass media or what have you. We may overcome our conditioning and patterns of behavior and remold ourselves consciously to that which we desire. We are not committed to a miserable future no matter how repressive our past has been.

This may sound optimistic. In one sense it is. Before this optimism is realized we need to have progressed beyond certain belief systems which many accept as dogma. Man is essentially free, he does not acknowledge or recognize this— this is our self-imposed limitation. Classical psychoanalysis has taught us that a portion of our being is essentially animal in nature. It is the striving for control of lower energies or animal nature that is responsible for the depressive illnesses which are so rampant and epidemic in our still egoistic society. Most of the time we are working with tremendous effort against ourselves. This struggle creates enormous mood shifts, the highs and the lows creating the illusion that external stimuli and control of external reality will create some type of happiness. We cannot expect to control all the forces in the world because there are too many with their own independent wills. We can only adapt and move with them.

What can be done, what can we do to help ourselves through and out of depression? An inspiration or a new idea will stimulate us, will put us into action. We create something to make us move out of this space. The problem in depression is the relative lack of energy and the blocking of any new or exciting thought forms. Thus, inspiration generally does not occur to a depressed person. Through a gradual process of nurturing, support, and mild coercion one may move into a different attitude. However, doctors can try to inspire the patient, thereby using medicine as a creative art.

How can this be achieved? By renewed sensitivity to the environment and the use of modalities which support and give vitality to our day-to-day existence. For example, art is lacking at most "mental" hospitals and other such institutions; the soul always responds to beauty—beauty is to the soul what food is to the body. For the most part, hospitals are the most negative, depressive, and sterile environments one comes into contact with. In mental hospitals the attitude prevails that people who wind up here are beyond help, and there is again the reliance upon drugs to create a change rather than human energy. Music, light, color, recreational therapy, sauna, hydrotherapy, yoga, tai chi—anything which creates a different mood can and should be employed to inspire those unfortunate beings who are suffering. We all possess the creativity, however suppressed, of potential artists. We need supportive development and patience. Dance therapy, yoga, massage, music, good food, fresh air, all administered by a generous, open, not overworked staff, will in time create a positive change in the most severely debilitated patient.

In treating depression we are dealing with but one of the many actors within us, and a change is possible regardless of what has happened in the past. It is the sense of futility, the caretaker attitude which persists on most wards of mental hospitals, which creates the reality. Those who deal with depressed, low-energy people must themselves be strong, positive vibrant people.

Drug therapy, the synthetic antidepressant, is *not* the answer. It must also be borne in mind that, first, nobody really knows how these drugs work and, second, the side effects often are disabling, creating subtle and not so subtle changes in human biochemistry.

It is interesting and a testimony to the blindness and arbitrariness of the lawmakers and medical authories that the best mood elevator known is considered an illegal drug. Marijuana is used by millions of Americans to elevate and change their feelings whenever it so pleases them. "Getting high" means allowing the vital energies to flow into conscious awareness. This herb has helped to create a social revolution and totally altered the belief structure of Western civilization. We in the medical profession deny ourselves this drug. There are few in the profession today who are not aware of the many possibilities this herb may have in alleviating emotional disturbances.

This herb is threatening because of its inherent ability to expand awareness. It allows for free thinking, self-realization for the moment, increased clarity, clarivoyance—it is a wonder drug and if used correctly and therapeutically can move this society closer to the goal of individual self-understanding.

Indian healing rituals both Eastern and Western have employed this drug or similar drugs throughout the centuries. We forbid ourselves this naturally occurring herb because of ridiculous self-imposed limitations as to what constitutes drug abuse. We do not know enough about it. Yet, there is probably no other drug that has been so extensively time-tested. We persist with high dosages of synthetic mood alternatives with known side effects.

Marijuana is not a panacea, however, it allows insight which can manifest as laughter, loss of anxiety, creative impulses, appreciation of light, color and sound. I have often heard interns, residents, and even senior medical men state that a patient needs a joint to calm him down. Marijuana is well-recognized as the finest anti-anxiety medication known to man.

Valium, Librium, and other tranquilizers are technology's answer for anxiety—its sales total in the billions. They are effective, however, they are also psychologically and physiologically addictive—they treat the symptoms not the source. Life appears to be a series of choices and once again collectively this society chooses synthetic medication to natural herbs.

Society today is beginning to question and reject technological medicine because technology is not responding to the searching, the longing, the pain which confronts and agonizes Western civilization.

Sound, Music and Color

The effect of sound on the physiology of the human body has been known scientifically for many years. It is believed that the tremendous incidence of hypertension in this country is party due to the high noise levels in cities. Sound is energy force and may create dissonance or resonance depending upon its frequency. The use of sound for military purposes stems back to the days of Jericho when Joshua used his trumpets to bring the walls down. The military has been experimenting with different frequencies of sound as weapons which can maim or destroy a person.

On the more positive side of things music and chanting have been used ritualistically by various cultures to alter consciousness and effect cures. The sound of the *Om* for example has been used for thousands of years in the East to clear the mind and bring serenity to the experiencer. Tibetan healing rites use high-pitched bells that create a clear sound which resonates with universal rhythms. These sounds create harmony and resonance; the vibrations enter into the aura (the electromagnetic field surrounding the body) and into and through the corporeal body.

The relationship of color and sound to health is extraordinary and certainly not coincidental when you realize there are seven notes, seven colors, seven chakras which relate to the seven glandular systems of the body, seven days of the week, and seven continents—*seven* is a mystical number. However, if we are bodies of electromagnetic energy it makes logical, scientific sense to consider ourselves subject to the laws of physics. The intelligent use of particular colors and sounds will positively influence us and change our energy state. What is potentially wonderful about this healing modality is that it overrides the intellectual aspect of personality and may allow you to experience aspects of yourself which you have been unconscious of.

It is interesting to note here a correlation of the potentialities of color for healing. The predominant color nature uses is green. On the visible color spectrum green is the fourth color which corresponds to the heart *chakra*. In metaphysics the color green represents Venus and the number "4" is the number of love. These relationships have been known for thousands of years in various advanced civilizations whose "medicine men" used color to heal. We are just becoming aware of the possibilities of such "unscientific" medical tools and I believe that the next 25 years will show a trememdous upsurge in research and experimental verification of the healing potentials of selected, modulated vibrations produced by color and music.

Music does soothe the savage soul. It is interesting to note the absence of music in most institutions. Pure harmonizing sound has the ability of putting us into the *Now*—we are taken up by the beauty of the music and the rational mind is shut off—we reach the state of pure receptivity. We are in the eternal moment, the Now. Because of clarity and beauty our minds and concentration are focused into the moment. The internal noise of the rational mind is shut down; we no longer live in the past, or future, or try to resolve things which have not happened, or try to correct things which happened in the past. Music can move us past ruminations, feelings of guilt, anger, self-punishment or any other negative emotion, can create for the moment self-realization—the recognition that we are *beings*. This happening occurs much more frequently than is commonly admitted and is often blocked because the ego is so strong that it will not permit the destruction of its limiting belief systems which keep us on a nonstop merry-go-round of disappointment and frustrations with occasional pleasures and triumphs.

The medical profession has been sold the idea that thorazine and the tricyclic antidepressants are the answers to controlling aberrant behavior, specifically schizophrenia and endogenous depression—these patients who suffer from withdrawal, contracted states are often subject to grotesque hallucinations, dangerous delusional states, illusions, confusion and an inability to effectively cope and function with life on a day-to-day basis. The orthodox medical model still does not explain and allow us to truly understand these bizarre behavioral patterns. Schizophrenia is still today a *dis*-ease which is ill-understood and an enigma to the medical profession. This is understandable because of the limitations of structured beliefs inculcated by medical schools which are suffering from illusion and delusion because their orthodox medical model does not recognize the existence of a soul or spirit. The key in dealing with this difficult medical problem lies in acceptance of the process of individual evolution—no two individuals experience the world the same way at the same period of time. We perpetually judge others by evaluating their behavior. This is valid but it is superficial; there exists much more beyond the world of appearances. The "problem" of schizophrenia opened up the medical profession to redefining reality. There are many, many "schizophrenic" people in the world who are able to deal effectively with their experiences. They have come to accept and integrate their experience as valid to themselves.

The healing profession needs to adopt the attitude of humility and acceptance to successfully deal with those who experience their world in a perhaps more profound, sensitive way. We need to create healing environments for the people unable to cope with a society which demands a high degree of a particular way of functioning. A person who undergoes a "psychotic break"—a sudden change in perception and concomitant mood—generally reacts with severe anxiety and fear. Any sudden change, particularly when it occurs in a nonsupportive atmosphere, can and does tear the individual asunder. To try to know the experience is impossible, it is unique to the experiencer. To empathize and to recognize that this possibility can exist within our own being is essential if rapport and meaningful help is to be given. To try to convince the person that what he is experiencing is not real, just imagination, is dangerous and superficial.

Most people have not consciously "allowed" or opened themselves up to altered states of consciousness. To negatively reinforce a painful, negative experience will create more pain and alienation; the depressed person will integrate the experience and his view of the world will take on a deeper more profound view. Hopefully, he will grow from the experience. To label a patient crazy is in a very real way labeling yourself as such because what is in front of you is a reflection of yourself. We can realize that we exist at different levels of experience which are relative to each other, constantly changing.

It is the static view of mechanistic philosophy which is so deadly and so wrong: We see an individual at a particular point in time and often that person is labeled and that person may be vulnerable enough to accept that concept of himself. We are all collectively responsible for the mentally imbalanced and chronically depressed. We do not want to recognize the reality that people with distorted views of the world exist. It is particularly distrubing that people with distorted perspectives on occasion have acquired enormous power and control!

Going *mad* is an understandably reactive process to a society which is increasingly more difficult to live in—the continuous paranoia, the poisoned, processed food, value systems and priorities which are nonhumanistic and drilled into us through an educational system which is increasingly out of touch with reality. But this process has given rise to the growth of psychotherapy, healing groups, counseling, and other modalities which are society's reaction to an increasingly unjustifiable, materialistic society, a society blinded by its own creations, the world of glamour, the world of technology gone past man's ability to handle his own imagination.

"We" created this world and it seems that a significant number of people see it as absurd, meaningless and painful. This pain which resides and is felt by everyone who allows himself to feel it is the collective ego. We are now in a profoundly "negative" point in our collective evolution. It is the collective health of ourselves which reflects this truth. There are approximately 10,000,000 alcoholics in this country, 2,000,000 women on the "pill" with all its attendant side effects, approximately 1,000,000 people on phenothiazine therapy, approximately one-third of the population clinically obese, an estimated 650,000 Americans contract cancer annually, a venereal disease epidemic, flu epidemics, suicide is one of the top ten causes of premature death in this country—it's a bleak picture. However, just as pain and suffering on an individual level create action in an attempt to ease and resolve the source of conflict, so will society collectively react to its collective pain and begin to recreate and reform a world which has become scarcely bearable. The emphasis must be on preventive medicine and environmental design has to be given top priority. The concept must be wholistic; healing and teaching must be emphasized. The creative imagination of the artist needs to be employed; technology must become our servant not our master.

6

The Drug Society

It is generally acknowledged that we are a nation of drug abusers. The extent of this abuse is a reflection of both an individual and a collective disharmony which we attempt to combat by using substances which hopefully will reestablish equilibrium via the relief of pain or by providing expansion of consciousness and insight to personal aspects which are generally hidden to everyday awareness and lie beyond ordinary reality.

Man suffers because of his addictions and conditioning which in themselves create predictable patterns of behavior. Predictable patterns of behavior are equated with stagnation and boredom which are the antitheses of inspiration. Growth means change and the breaking down of limitations and attitudes which create a sense of separation and duality. There is no duality. There is only one thing going on within the universe and that one thing is a conscious living mental energy which comprises and moves all things. The illusion of separateness is the creator of pain because it blocks communication and the flow of energy. To help ease our pain and abolish our loneliness we seek out help in the form of medications or herbs to help release us from our inhibitions (programmed memory traces) and behavior which create feelings of isolation, withdrawal, loneliness, and fear. We have within ourselves the ability to experience true freedom in our own way and within our own means. We have the power to evolve, and this involves the conscious awareness that we are all unique aspects of a living, growing, evolving universe. As we learn to freely communicate and express ourselves we move toward balance, health and happiness.

The extraordinary abuse of drugs, illicit or legal, is a reflection of the inner and outer anxieties and stress generated by a society which collectively imposes a value and priority system in opposition to the basic desires and aspirations of the individual. We have deluded ourselves as to what constitutes a drug and have imposed severe limitations on what an individual may ingest into his body, acting from the concept that we know what is essentially good for one and not good for another. However, the law of supply and demand is working at all times and people will get what they ask for. What does this mean in regards to the national schizophrenia regarding the drug "problem?" It means a growing awareness of the attempts by "authorities" to suppress these substances which we lump together as "drugs." This attitude has created an enormous polarity of forces characterized by moralists and bureaucrats attempting to deny fundamental human rights.

We tyrannize ourselves with a dehumanized educational system and false priorities, and as we witness an unprecedented national health catastrophy we try to remedy the situation not by compassion and understanding but by a mind-boggling array of synthetic chemicals which more often than not create further internal disequilibriums. Many, if not most, of these prescription drugs act in a manner which is unknown and symptomatic at best; we refuse to recognize or are unable to see that the ingestion of large doses of any foreign substance will work against us and our bodily processes because they are simply attempts to cover up an underlying malady. We look to medical technology for salvation. This is a blind deceit. We have to recognize that our health is our own responsibility and we must do those things which contribute to our welfare and sense of well-being rather than those which detract from it.

We need to see the drug problem clearly in the light of subjective as well as objective data, recognizing the right of the individual to explore various modalities which may help him along the road to self-understanding and health. I believe that drugs are not necessary for the establishment of health, however, the proper, responsible, and ritualistic use of various mind-expanding agents such as LSD, mescaline and psilocybin have enormous *potential* in the growth process.

Various hallucinogens and euphoria producers were used in ancient divination rites as well as in helping unfortunate individuals locked into a particularly unpleasant aspect of their subconscious mind. If a human being can perceive the intense beauty of his true being for however short a period of time, then we have done something to ameliorate suffering and added to our own well-being. A society which is product-oriented, as opposed to process-oriented, feels threatened by its own structure. Puritan morality is deeply imbedded within the collective subconscious of this culture and, it is dying a slow, painful death.

There is nothing wrong with being "high." Being high is feeling good and only a masochist enjoys misery. Any agent or technique which is effective in elevating spirit and health is valid be it dancing, singing, laughing or getting stoned.

The national drug problem is not due to the abuse or indulgence of marijuana, LSD, cocaine, or even heroin. The national drug problem is alcohol, barbiturates, steroids, aspirins, tranquilizers, nicotine, caffeine, phenothiazines, and antihypertensive medications. These are the opiates of the masses and poor choices indeed for prolonged use of these agents will create sustained, systemic disease manifestations.

Why is it that we spend so much time and effort to disapprove the use of "illegal" drugs and do not recognize the iatrogenic disasters which confound and confront any practicing physician who indulges in the issuing of proprietary synthetic medications?

The reaction to this obvious dichotomy has created, particularly in young people, a "healthy" skepticism of the medical profession and yet many people with real medical problems are left with few alternatives. This progressive loss of faith in orthodox medicine is real and has created the atmosphere responsible for the medical malpractice crisis. The malpractice crisis may be seen as a reaction by the people to a system of medicine which is not providing adequate relief. From this frustration and lack of relief from pain ensued vindictive attitudes towards the profession which professes to help them in a meaningful way. The medical profession has deluded itself in propagandizing its own potency, not wanting to recognize its severe limitations and not wanting to look at and examine the iatrogenic disasters which befall most practicing doctors.

What people are looking for are alternatives—safe, effective agents or therapies which are understandable and not clouded in ambiguous medical jargon and ritual which only create misunderstanding and apprehension. We need to seek out and develop the natural therapies in which the emphasis is on self-healing and self-reliance. This is an enormous task for our educational process needs to be redirected and reoriented for both the lay public and the helping and healing professions.

Western medicine's emphasis is disease or pathology oriented. A diagnosis is entertained and confirmed by various tests and a drug regime is developed. The overdependence on drugs is both superficial and symptomatic as the real power of drugs lies in the suggestive effect which is transferred from doctor to patient. The problem, however, is not in the transference itself but in the incredible array of unwanted effects upon the physiology of the body which so many of these agents create. The positive suggestion or placebo effect is often overridden by the real physiologic damage incurred by many of today's modern "therapeutic" agents. As long as we deal on such a superficial plane the problem simply will not go away; the real causation of *dis*ease resides within the psyche or thinking mechanism of the individual. Healthy mind, healthy body—this movement away from pathology to self-responsibility for health reaches fruition when you begin to perceive the true relationship within yourself and your immediate environment.

At this point we have created an artificial separation of "good" versus "bad" drugs. We should realize that which is "good" or "bad" is based upon our own experience. We all have unique personalities and unique metabolic systems which are determined genetically and thereby react to drugs or herbs in their own way. As long as medicine is practiced in a standardized, inflexible manner and refuses to recognize the sensitivity and uniqueness of the individual then it is doomed to limited success and inadequacy. The problem resides in the dichotomy of what we have professed we can do and understand as opposed to what we really can do and what we really do not understand. The more the public recognizes and knows the limitations of modern medicine the less it will be angered when the standard surgical and medical therapies fall short of what is claimed.

We have assumed too much responsibility, living the illusion inculcated into us in medical school, of the power and effectiveness of medical science. True science is based upon the observation of nature. Science gets distorted when a scientist does not want to recognize that that which he predicts as a potential outcome does not in actuality occur. In other words, we need to reevaluate scientifically the failures of most of our therapeutic modalities and attempt to discover the laws of nature which govern health.

We have abdicated our bodies and minds to technologies and sciences which deal essentially with objective data. Medical science cannot explain the subjective or intuitive world which lies beyond quantification, beyond intellectualization, beyond verification, beyond documentation and standardization. It is unique to each of us. God, life, energy, spirit, or superconsciousness is behind all manifestation and yet we cannot prove its existence except through our own direct experience of it. The power of science and the power of the intellect are real but they are only relative, and an over-reliance on another person's interpretation of reality is placing oneself above or below another human being. As the universe is an expanding intelligence we need to realize that there are greater and lesser degrees of understanding within this dynamic universe but that all these intelligences derive their life and sustenance from the same source. It is for this reason that doctors, gurus or whoever, must be demystified and put into proper perspective.

The medical profession is doing a service for mankind— we have the power to alleviate pain. We have the tools to do this. We also have the power to create pain and disease. It is the nature and the degree of understanding which we employ which determines the relative success or failure of our therapeutic undertaking. The more we rely on our own judgment and feelings the greater the possibility of being effective and clear.

Drugs are a *tool*, they can be lifesaving, life-giving; they can also be our detractors and destroyers. A rule of thumb is that moderation is the best approach and that large amounts of drugs in themselves create side effects which immediately negate the initial intention of taking such an agent. In other

words it makes no sense to take a drug to relieve one symptom only to create another symptom. Sounds ridiculous.
However, this problem occupies a great deal of time in clinical medicine today. The lack of real belief in many of the
doctors who employ such medications create a functional
"schizophrenia" in that the doctor feels obliged to somehow
or other treat the patient with something and yet is not con-
vinced of the real worth of many of today's therapeutic
regimes. He is also obliged morally and legally to do his best
to help relieve the patient's duress and does the best he can
with what is available. It is a time of change and we need to
recognize the truth that many of us have become slaves to
technology and synthetic compounds. Drugs should be our
servants not our masters; to be used wisely and reasonably.

Alcohol

Alcoholic abuse is the number one drug problem in the
United States today. There are an estimated 10,000,000 alcoholics presently living in this country. The cost and social
ramifications of chronic alcoholism is truly astounding—if
you look at both the obvious and subtle effects of alcoholic
abuse you may see how this drug has helped to rip apart the
fabric of this society.

We are all aware of the disasters which alcohol creates
over the long term, be it personal, family, or involving the in-
juring and death of innocent people. We are also aware that
at least half of all auto deaths are caused by intoxication; the
disruptive effects upon the family are well-documented; the
cost to the economy in terms of inefficiency, working days
lost, and sloppy workmanship are all common knowledge.

The problems of the alcoholic are individual and yet one
may see this move toward alcoholic abuse as but an example
of how an individual reacts to his own conditioning and
reflects it back upon his family and immediate society. Our

life is our own responsibility and we learn through a process of trial and error that the creation and cause of this "problem" resides within our ability to successfully integrate and gain control of our own emotions. We constantly seek relief from pain and anxiety, and the alcoholic abuse in this society is but a manifestation of the collective imbalance that is all about us daily.

Alcohol abuse is the result of a negative perception of self, lack of self-esteem and the inability to successfully cope with inner drives and interpersonal relationships. Its use and abuse is an attempt to experience good feelings within and thereby be able to relate in a more flowing or harmonic way with friends, family, and associates. The problem with alcohol is that it opens up negative as well as positive aspects of our personality but still hides from our conscious awareness the possibility of really knowing ourselves. The alcoholic characteristically suffers from a poor self-image, and sees himself as a failure. The alcoholic drinks to change his "normal" perception of reality which is but a projection of his negative programming and egotistical manifestations.

Our limited perception creates impositions and limitations upon ourselves. These limitations are acted out in the lower self—the ego waging war against the higher self. We seek solace from our pain and get drunk so that we may forget the grinding reality of boredom, noncommunication, and aloneness. This aloneness and feelings of isolation are the paramount features of the alcoholic world and are a result of a conditioning process which has been imprinted from early childhood into the subconscious mind. The inability to transcend and grow beyond our conditioning results in extreme pain and suffering and ultimately leads to self-destruction.

The fate of the alcoholic may assume many unhappy possibilities: bleeding to death from esophageal varices, the agony of cirrhosis of the liver, nerve and brain damage, muscle wasting, the loss of the will to live. It's a nasty way out yet a very popular one. There is a point of no return where attitudes and beliefs are so fixed and jaundiced that any amount of preaching, lecturing or begging will not stir the alcoholic to action; behind the facade lies a soul who experiences deep psychic pain, fear, bitterness, and confusion.

The alcoholic may see the world as a cruel paradox, a meaningless experience and thereby rationalize his attitude and behavior by escaping into an even more distorted view of reality. Alcohol is a depressant and only in very high doses does one occasionally glimpse the subconscious reality which may appear as vivid hallucinations, however, the personality has usually disintegrated and these experiences are not recognized as significant.

Alcohol abuse is but a symptomatic cure for temporarily changing behavior. It does not bring the individual into himself where he may be able to examine and explore the anxieties which are creating turmoil and torment. Alcohol is not a consciousness expanding drug; it releases from normal control lower forces and drives which in time destroy the functioning of the body.

Education and rehabilitation are the key to its treatment. The alcoholic industry should subsidize the hospitals and treatment centers. A great percentage of hospital beds today are filled by individuals who are suffering from alcohol related problems such as ulcers, cirrhosis, pancreatitis, organic brain syndromes, various neuropathies, impotence, general debility, heart failure, malnutrition, obesity, auto accidents, child abuse, and trauma due to physical violence.

Amphetamines

These are synthetic amines which act with a pronounced stimulant effect on the central nervous system. It is believed that they potentiate the effects of the sympathetic nervous system. Its medical uses today consist of treating a syndrome called *narcolepsy* which is characterized by an inability to stay awake. Also, amphetamines are used empirically in hyperactive children where the drug has a paradoxical effect to that found in adults; in hyperactive children the drug exerts a calming effect upon the children. Amphetamines were widely used for the control of obesity, however, its addictive nature and undesirable side effects have made this mode of therapy unpopular for both physician and patient alike.

As these drugs increase the energy level it is understandable why they have been so abused. It is another attempt to use high doses of external agents to change feelings. This creates in itself an imbalance as it accents and stimulates the sympathetic nervous system; it momentarily deranges the normal homeostatic mechanisms of the body which will re-equilibrate after the drug effect wears off. The drug creates a temporary feeling of power, alertness, and excitement which is short-lived and if you enjoy that level of consciousness then you will desire to experience it again and again.

Amphetamines are but another dangerous attempt to create a different reality; they are but another choice where the individual must weigh the advantages and disadvantages of rapid mood shifts. The danger lies in the individual's inability to gain a desired conscious control over his own behavior patterns. The other danger of amphetamines lies in their chronic use. The drug appears to be capable of creating permanent damage to the brain itself.

Barbiturates

These synthetic central nervous system depressant drugs were initially used to induce sleep. If used in small doses they are effective in relieving tension and anxiety and, like tranquilizers, do not cause excessive drowsiness. In larger doses their selective benefit is lost, while their depressant actions spread to all parts of the central nervous system and spinal cord. A barbiturate-induced sleep resembles natural sleep *except* that a distrubance of the rapid eye movement (R.E.M.) has been noted which indicates the sleep rhythm is impaired, which suggests that subtle psychological conseqúences may occur. It is becoming increasingly understood how sound sleep is vital to the consciousness and health of an individual. Deep relaxed sleep affords opportunity for your consciousness to explore and communicate in the world of the "collective unconscious" where one directly experiences and communicates in a reality far different and removed from that of the conscious, objective world.

The inability to sleep and the problem of insomnia reflect conflict, anxiety, and tension which have not been normally dissipated. There are many non-drug techniques available today, especially those dealing with rhythmic breathing, which will induce relaxation and deep sleep. Autohypnosis or autosuggestion is one of the most effective forms of self-relaxation. You "program" yourself through suggestion to systematically relax various parts of the body through selective contraction and relaxation of various muscle groups. However, this takes personal effort—motivation, and understanding of the process, practice, and an awareness of the higher aspects of consciousness. The majority of Americans would rather reach for a pill to temporarily resolve the inherent problem of living. The problem with this approach is that these synthetic drugs upset the internal mechanisms of the body, create many allergic reactions and are exquisitely habit forming. There is also the problem of tolerance which creates a need to take progressively larger doses of the medication to induce a comparable physiological effect as the drug induces metabolic enzymes within the liver to assist in its detoxification.

The extraordinary abuse of these substances but again reflect a society in conflict with itself; the inability to find peace within oneself and the reliance on external agents for palliation.

Many people are not aware of the addictive nature of such substances and the agonies of barbiturates withdrawal are more serious than heroin withdrawal. (I may add here that the "horrors" of heroin withdrawal have been greatly exaggerated through dramatic presentations and in no way compare with the physiological nightmares created by large doses of barbiturates or alcohol.) Withdrawal symptoms closely resemble the delirium tremens of the alcoholic and include weakness, violent tremors, anxiety, increased temperature, rapid pulse, violent epileptic-like seizures. By the third day psychoses resembling schizophrenia with paranoid delusions and vivid hallucinations may develop. This is no innocuous drug. Barbiturates are the number one drug of choice for suicide attempts, successful and unsuccessful.

Caffeine

The drug caffeine is a stimulant of the central nervous system. One cup of coffee contains approximately 150 mgs of caffeine. Generally caffeine induces feelings of alertness and well-being, exhilaration, or euphoria. Onset of fatigue, inattentiveness, boredom, and sleepiness is postponed. Excessive prolonged consumption of caffeine causes anxiety, tremors, insomnia, restlessness, headaches, and confusion. Coffee in excess will stimulate gastric secretion and exacerbate peptic ulcers.

Cocaine

One of the favorite drugs of the counterculture, particularly those people in the artistic world. Its popularity is due to its ability to change the level of energy; this drug derived from coca leaves enhances both mental and physical awareness.

The rush of energy turns the individual "on"; he is tapping into that infinite reservoir of energy which is available to us at any time. As stated in the *Qabalah*, a philosophic doctrine based upon the esoteric interpretation of the Bible, "All the power that ever was or will be is here now."

This anesthetic appears to shut down the rational scanning mind which consistently keeps us in a state of distraction and disharmony. It allows you to come into direct communication with your higher faculties and, depending upon the personality and will, enables you to direct energy however you please. This herb/drug opens you up to the higher centers and you can feel the incredible rush of energy course through your body. You become aware of yourself— the physical/mental jolt enhances inherent creativity and sensuality. Cocaine's real appeal stems from its ability to enhance the sexual experience to levels which are otherwise beyond the reach of normal sexual indulgences.

We are receivers and transmitters of energy; our brains are similar to step-up or step-down transformers and as we open up to the subconscious energies, be it through meditative techniques or by using certain drugs as catalysts, we are allowing ourselves to directly experience the pure consciousness of our inner selves. It is as if a veil has been pulled away and the energies of the universe are directly perceived and experienced. The quality of the altered state of awareness is unique to each individual. However, cocaine is a stimulant to the central nervous system and its addictive nature lies not in its pharmacology but in its ability to elicit excitation and pleasurable sensual gratification. As in anything else, these feelings and moods are deemed desirable when compared to other more mundane perceptions of reality. The cocaine experience falls into the positive side of the Yin-Yang equilibrium and the depression often reported by cocaine users is a result of a drop in energy and a moving back into a different, less intense feeling and flow.

Cocaine's popularity in this culture is understandable as this is a speed culture, a culture which enjoys sensation, power and action. Cocaine was used extensively by Sigmund Freud and his extensive preoccupation with sexual fantasy could be equated with the knowledge that cocaine will induce extraordinary sexual experiences on the physical plane. You can really let go with this drug; the inhibitions (the super-ego) and the ego defenses collapse with the entry into aspect of reality of which most people are unconscious. This herb has been used extensively, everyday and ritualistically, by the indians of Peru and Bolivia.

A parallel anesthetic which induces similar transcending experiences is nitrous oxide, laughing gas. One of the definitive essays regarding human consciousness and man's relationship to the cosmos can be found in William James' *Varieties of Religious Experience.* His experience was derived from the use of nitrous oxide. My personal experience involved a similar anesthetic called *LiDoCaine*, legally and medically induced. I was having some surgery done on my finger and the local anesthetic was given via an intravenous block. A tourniquet was wrapped above the site of the medication and when the operation was finished the tourniquet was released. I suddenly felt flushed with a marvelous exhilaration and the overhead flood lamp suddenly burst forth in marvelous colors. I started laughing riotously as if my psyche's funny bone had been simulated. The experience was immediately terminated by a quick-acting barbiturate which brought me back down. My behavior was not only inappropriate but frightening to the anesthesiologist who could not relate to the experience. It was a meaningful, delightful experience, a glimpse into the joyous cosmology of which we are all a part.

Cocaine's danger lies not in the user's physical dependence or tolerance but in the strong psychic dependence due to the extreme mood elevations, elation, and power which may be experienced. The drug facilitates moving to another level or vibrational state which is more exciting, intense, and conscious than the state which preceded it. It allows one to concentrate and focus energies which alter perception and thereby raise the consciousness. The resultant depression is a result of the change in energy state. The natural feeling is a disappointment. Self-image suffers as you return to your "old self" which is a product of your conditioning, habits, and patterns of behavior.

Cocaine as do other drugs bypass the arduous process otherwise necessary to reach the reality of the higher self. The problem with the experience is that in time its excitement fades and one recognizes the need for equilibration— *Peace.* The intensity with which this drug is sought is but another indication of man's eternal need to find himself and experience freedom from his self-imposed limitations and conditioning.

This drug/herb is far down the morbidity list when compared to substances such as alcohol, barbiturates, and nicotine. It is a threat to the authorities and moralists of our society in that people who take this and similar drugs very often undergo a profound change in attitude and belief about themselves and the society in which they find themselves. This creates an obvious threat to the power of the "authorities" and the "establishment."

Prosecution for use of this drug, as with any other drug, is an infringement upon personal rights. Each and every one of us has a God-given right to live the life we so choose even if it appears from the perspective of others to be morally bankrupt, decadent, or whatever. As the society matures so will its attitudes toward drugs and herbs; through experience hopefully we will learn to use these substances judiciously and with respect for their power and potential for real growth. The decision to use or not use drugs is an individual one and the individual must assume responsibility for his/her actions.

Phenothiazines

This drug was introduced in the early 1950s. Its major use is for the control of psychotic behavior and treatment of schizophrenia. Its evolution is interesting as it was initially hailed as the answer for schizophrenia—a complex mental dis-ease characterized by disorders of feeling, of conduct and of thought, and an increasing withdrawal of interest from the world.

In 1911, Paul Bleuler introduced the term *schizophrenia*. Bleuler considered the fundamental symptoms to be disturbances of association and affectivity, a prediliction for fantasy as against reality (whose reality?) and a tendency to divorce from reality. Hallucinations, delusions, illusions, and catatonic symptoms he called secondary symptoms while conceding that these were the symptoms which often made manifest the psychosis and caused the patient to be hospitalized.

There has been little advance in the classification of schizophrenia since Emil Kraeplin and Paul Bleuler; their descriptive work has not been superceded. Kraeplin and Bleuler believed that schizophrenia was the outcome of a pathological, anatomical, or chemical disturbance of the brain. To this date this etiology has not been successfully proven.

Adolf Meyer adopted a different view. The essence of his view was that schizophrenia is the outcome of progressive maladaptation of the individual to his environment. He stated that schizophrenia is not a *disease* but a congeries of individual types of reactions having certain general similarities.

Meyer concluded that schizophrenia is the end result of an accumulation of faulty habits of *reaction*—the person withdraws, becomes alienated from himself and society and thereby cuts himself off from communication. His world view is often hostile, negative and fearful. He may see the world as hostile and working against him and thereby blame "others" for his "failures." As he retreats into himself he becomes introspective and the mind creates, real or imagined, delusional, illusional systems of thought which are quite painful, and often terrifying. He does not love himself, nor is he capable of loving another. This break from real communication creates a blocking of energy which creates altered states of consciousness that are particularly unpleasant. The experiencer is seeing reality from a negative aspect and suffering from this distorted view of reality. The artist may see and feel things which are beyond that of the average person just as the schizophrenic. However, his inability to communicate these feelings to others create isolation and withdrawal. The reaction of others to this different view of reality often leads to greater distress and frustration; their lack of understanding and guidance reinforces his negative self-image and his behavior may or may not manifest unpleasant or negative traits. However, once we realize that within each of us lies the potential to manifest any type of behavior and/or thought, then we must take a look again at those who are social outcasts and live on the fringes of society. Perhaps their only "sin" has been their inability to adapt to a sociocultural structure which is increasingly absurd and distorted, complex and confusing. This maladaptation, if not accepted or understood by the individual himself, will create and engender feelings of isolation, loneliness, and misery.

Freud's explanation of schizophrenia centered around the problem of the ego. In his view the primary process in schizophrenia is a profound unconscious mental regression and turning inwards with the withdrawal of libido (desire) from reality, its objects and relationships. This regression may be precipitated by emotional traumata or conflicts of various kinds, and is particularly apt to occur at critical periods of biological development; it is facilitated by some earlier trauma in the development and organization of the ego which has caused a fixation at a more immature level of autoeroticism or narcissism. Contacts with reality are progressively lost as the illness develops and the ego, reinvested with its libido, becomes again egocentric and narcissistic. The abandonment of relations with reality and the withdrawal of libido (interest, desire) from objects lead to the development of feelings of depersonalization and derealization, and to such delusions as those of the death of relatives or of world destruction.

While there are many theories as to the etiology of schizophrenia today there is no concrete evidence as to an exact causation of this type of behavior. What is important to understand is that the nature of reality is a highly subjective statement, made as a direct result of personal beliefs, attitudes, and reactions. There is reality and there is *reality*. One deals with the machinations and melodramas of the self or ego which continually sees itself in a world of subject/object, us-versus-them, and acts out of reaction and not under the conscious influence of the higher self.

Reality, for me, acknowledges the concept of the higher self or the "I Am" which brings the lower self under its conscious control; the personality comes to know that it always has been an extension of the "I Am," which till that point had been caught in the illusion of *otherness*. Everything that is going on is going on *now* and therein lies an infinite variety of manifestations, behaviors, thoughts and actions which are continuously in a state of change. To quantitate, to classify, to objectify, to moralize is only to miss the point because reality lies beyond judgment; in the end you can only judge yourself. The problems begin when other people react to our behavior and deem it undesirable. This is not to say that society should not and will not protect itself from individuals who act out negative behavior patterns. But as people begin to see the commonablity of all experience then society is less apt to react in a fashion which is oppressive and destructive toward those individuals who are having difficulties in their own personal evolution.

There are people who are more aware, advanced, loving

than others; but all of us must realize that we are all living within our *own* process and are at a particular point of evolution, and then there is danger in taking measures, particular chemical, surgical or shock measures to control or supress behavior which we cannot rationalize or understand. What medical science does not want to recognize is the existence of soul or spirit and to realize that the real struggle of man is to merge with his higher nature which he experiences as progressive feelings of well-being, health, and happiness.

When society recognizes those in need and attempts to nurture them back to health and sanity, the problem resides not in the intentions but in the methods of trying to correct or ameliorate such behavior. The methods have "progressed" from prefrontal lobotomies to electroconvulsive therapy to phenothiazines which I view as a form of "chemical lobotomy." This drug has its place in the initial treatment of persons whose behavior is totally out of control, however, long-term treatment with this modality interferes and blocks growth and the thinking process.

The standard approach to control negative experiences and behavior is to place a person in a mental hospital and/or administer phenothiazines. Chlorpromazine, a phenothiazine derivative is used extensively in this country to control behavior. Its extensive use currently is being critically examined. Why? First, its action is not understood. Second, its use is being directed toward personality states, such as schizophrenia, which have not been understood within the present conceptual medical model. Essentially, we have been using a chemical modality of uncertain action for a disease syndrome which is ill-understood!

What is wrong with phenothiazines? The January 1976 issue of the *American Journal of Psychiatry* posed the interesting question, "Is the *cure* worse than the dis-ease?" The initial faith with which this drug was first introduced into the medical profession and its subsequent history outlines the growing evolution of human understanding. It has moved, in the course of 25 years, from that of an answer for schizophrenia to that of a superficially dangerous attempt to change or control that which we do not fully understand. The side effects are many and may be serious and long-term treatment with phenothiazines creates a syndrome of persistent *tardive dyskinesia*, a clinical manifestation of the poisoning and destruction of portions of the brain that coordinate and maintain smooth functioning of the muscular systems of the body. It is now known that irreversible dyskinesia may result from prolonged use, the presumption being that the damage is secondary to desctruction of the basal ganglion in the brain. This persistent dyskinesis has been well-delineated by Hunter and his colleagues (1974) who found 15 of these cases (6 percent) in a group of 250 patients who have been treated in a mental hospital for more than 18 months with phenothiazines. All were women over the age of 55 and demented due to brain damage from other causes—following leucotomy or electroconvulsive therapy or a result of senile or arteriosclerotic brain disease. The dyskinesia had developed insidiously and usually secondarily to drug-induced Parkinsonism. There was continual and distressing grimacing and contorting of the face with writhing, chewing, sucking and gaping movements of the mouth, tongue and jaws, Rapid protrusion and withdrawal of the tongue may interfere with eating and drinking, speech may become hoarse and even unintelligible and sudden closure of the glottis may precipitate respiratory distress. These abnormal movements of the face region are frequently accompanied by agitation (akathisia) and minor choreiform movements of the limbs. They are not relieved by anti-Parkinsonian drugs and persist after the phenothiazines are withdrawn.

Additionally there is acute photosensitivity in summer with redness and edema of the exposed skin which a few patients show. More significant oculocutaneous lesions may develop in patients treated with phenothiazines, particularly chlorpromazine in high dosage over a long period. Eye changes usually precede changes in skin pigmentation. Lesions of the lens have been recorded in a quarter to one-third of patient samples, and in at least a quarter of these affected individuals there have been corneal lesions also. Fortunately these changes, though persistent, are seldom disabling, visual acuity apparently only rarely being impaired. The viscera also may become pigmented during treatment with phenothiazines, and it is possible that in some cases cardiac damage results; a few patients have died suddenly and unexpectedly when under treatment with these drugs, and there often has been little or no evident cause for this discovered at postmortem examination. Studying 4,000 patients treated with phenothiazines, Ayd (1961) found that 21 percent had akathisia (agitation), 15 percent Parkinsonism and over 2 percent dystonic movements.

The evidence against phenothiazines is now incontrovertible, but there are some who definitely feel that this drug still has therapeutic advantages. However from my perspective I can never justify a medication which intrinsically damages organic areas of the brain. To summarize the difficulties and subtleties of clinical medicine particularly when one's own personal belief system is brought into question, I offer the following interchange which occurred with a meeting of psychiatrists concerning drug abuse.

Dr. X: "When we give patients drugs for suppressing emotional symptoms, are we really treating them or are we merely subduing them because we don't want to deliver human services? Whom are we servicing when we administer psychotrophic drugs? Society, which gives us a mandate to take care of people at low cost? Are we serving the patient—or ourselves as professionals who want to believe we are doing something for the patient? Or, do we just want to make it easier for ourselves?

"In talking about the right to treatment, a fashionable topic today, many infer that being given a drug such as thorazine is a right rather than a police action to control and quiet a patient. Many physicians claim that drugs are the real therapeutic modality in state mental hospitals; that drugs are responsible for "cures," for getting people discharged, for emptying the back wards. Well, I don't agree . . .

"Some of my patients do take drugs, but they don't get them from me. I don't object if they want medication and they go to a physician, who is in a better position to give a physical exam and to oversee drug reactions than I am.

"But I must say that when a patient is on drugs, particularly the major tranquilizers and antidepressants, and come into my office, I can spot it immediately. The patient doesn't relate, doesn't communicate as previously. He may no longer talk about delusions or hallucinations, but he'll no longer talk about anything else pertinent either."

With these remarks pandemonium erupted. Several psychiatrists simultaneously protested and attested to their belief in the therapeutic efficacy of drugs:

"At least drugs can offer a person in misery some relief," declared one. "At least depressed patients on antidepressants can return to some functioning. Many return to an active, productive life; many become quite able to enjoy themselves."

"When used properly, these drugs are extremely valuable therapeutic agents," injected another.

"It's a matter of the functions we ascribe to these drugs and how we as physicians use them," asserted a third. "Correctly used, they have definite value for the patient."

In parrying the barrage of protests Dr. X insisted: "It's the same as drinking or smoking cigarettes. When I smoked, I was aware that the cigarettes had an enormous tranquilizing effect. I don't believe that we as physicians should go about promoting a drug culture as a solution to a person's agony."

Whereupon another speaker protested Dr. X's "indis-

criminantly lumping together phenothiazines, alcohol, cigarettes and minor tranquilizers."

The preceding dialogue indicates the changing tide of
opinion as regards this controversial subject. Ultimately we
can only base our decision after carefully analyzing the data.
From the standpoint of personal human ecology, any substance which creates so many side effects is of limited or no
value.

The following case history illustrates the predicament in
which a psychiatrist or medical practitioner finds himself. A
young man, age 22, entered my office complaining of severe
anxiety. His major complaint was that he was suffering from
auditory hallucinations; when he came in he was very excited, his pupils were dilated, and he was sweating profusely.

A startling phenomenon had occurred to this young
man. He had always aspired to be a musician, however, he
had experienced no inspiration up to this point in his life.
Suddenly, without explanation this man's perception of
reality changed dramatically, he began to consciously experience music. He was receiving sudden illumination and
inspiration from his higher nature. Obviously, he had a
tremendous immediate reversal of self-image. He was consciously experiencing the creative aspect of himself. On
further examination he showed me a book filled with
music which he had written; he was in a hyperkinetic state
and was unable to sleep. He could not believe what was
happening to him, yet it really was! He had become very
sensitive to both positive and negative feelings and found
the city overwhelming. He had experienced similar episodes while under the influence of LSD-25, however, this
event was spontaneous. All he really wanted and needed
was support and guidance to let him know that it was all
right. He knew this intellectually, however, he doubted
himself and found it difficult to accept that such a miraculous creative process could occur to *him*. How another

doctor or psychiatrist would have reacted to such a situation is problematic, the fact that he was integrating the experience into positive expression would suggest that he would not require or benefit from drug therapy. However, often times in the process of unfoldment a man may get in touch with painful emotions which he cannot understand and integrate and his internalization of them creates fear and anxiety. In this situation, he would be an obvious target for phenothiazine or similar drug which in time would cause him to abnegate his newfound creativity.

Tar and Nicotine

The problem of cigarette addiction as in other addictions is rooted within the psyche of the person. The ritual's power lies within its ability to reduce stress and anxiety. The problems attendant to cigarette smoking are complex in that there is so strong an association between smoking and lung and heart disease. The idea or suggestion that cigarette smoking is inherently bad for one's health creates in itself the attendant fear and guilt which are prerequisite to the eventual outcome of death.

Nicotine in itself creates a sympathetic stimulation of the cardiovascular system. There is vasoconstriction of the skin and vasodilatation in the muscles, tachycardia and a rise in the blood pressure of approximately 15 mm mercury systolic and 10 mm mercury diastolic. Ventricular extrasystoles may occur. Cardiac output, work and oxygen consumption increase. The effect of cigarette smoke on the lungs reduces the lungs' capacity to extract oxygen. The primary causation or pathogenesis of cancer is due to decreased oxygen levels at the cellular level. This physiological effect working in conjunction with the suggestions that cigarette smoking causes lung cancer and heart disease will in itself impose neurochemical impulses which will create the arterial spasm and decreased oxygen perfusion to the tissues, with the resultant possibility that those areas where flow is decreased will necrose and undergo malignant change. Such is the power of the mind.

Self-hypnosis is an extremely effective technique in relieving the desire for smoking and works through subconsciousness to break the reactive type of behavior which is seen in compulsive smokers. Once again we need to be aware of why we are doing what we are doing and take constructive action to change unwanted behavior.

Heroin

This growing tragedy is rooted within the psyche of this nation; so many of our young people are finding the educational system to be irrelevant or meaningless and the inability to find meaningful work or to find work at all are probably the major reasons why so many young people are turning to this deadly substance—to withdraw and try to forget about a world which they see in terms of confusion, pain, and loneliness. The lack of work creates boredom, futility, and often desperation. Boredom is the antithesis to creativity and creativity is a fundamental desire among human beings. There is a knowingness, consciously or subconsciously, that we are responsible to the collective society and thereby need to contribute to it.

Morphine, from which heroin is derived, is a drug which has been used for centuries to produce a dream-like euphoria, traditionally it has been either smoked or used as snuff. It is estimated that approximately half of the English aristocracy in the 1800s were using morphine regularly. This is but another indication of man's relentless desire to transcend himself.

Today we see the resultant phenomenon of heroin addiction. It is not taken in moderate doses and it is injected directly into the blood stream, creating an initial exquisite high. However, this effect wears off in time and the addict is faced with an enormous physical craving. Without the peak experience the heroin then becomes an agent to relieve the pain of the addiction. The subcultural aspects of the addict's world have been brought to the public eye through crime, particularly prostitution and mugging—the intensity of the desire is enormous, the human suffering is inestimatable. All one has to do is visit a city emergency room and look at what is going on.

The most tragic case I have ever seen was a young girl who was pregnant, her body wasted, her arms shredded with track marks, her face somber and sunken and her teeth destroyed. She came to the emergency room to see if she could get false teeth; she was a prostitute and her appeal was diminished by her crumbling appearance. Yet, behind all this were eyes that were clear and I could still see the dwindling sparkle of youth which was being steadily diminished by her addiction.

Society's answer to date has been to use another synthetic drug called *methadone*, substituting one poison for another. The rational being that it keeps the addicts off the street. But it also continues the addiction while slowly destroying the person's health. What are the solutions to this problem? We need to see these unfortunate people for what they are—people who are trapped in a vicious cycle in that they are addicted to a substance which is deemed illegal by society. And yet, in an objective view of things, we cannot really say that heroin is any worse than the alcohol or barbiturate problem. The problem is that it is illegal and hence a black market item with all the attendant problems. People will always find a way to get what they want.

Our choices are really threefold: 1) we can continue to use methadone, which is a toxic, addicting substance in itself, used in a superficial treatment program which does not heal; 2) legalize the heroin and at the same time have massive rehabilitation and education programs; 3) develop supportive drug detoxification centers, preferably in the countryside where addicts can go to do work, detoxify, and be supported in an atmosphere where there is appropriate use of herbs, clean water, sunlight, exercise, and rest.

The third alternative is obviously the compassionate answer. The first is the expedient answer and the second recognizes the reality of the situation and mass hypocrisy regarding drug use in this country. Once again, we need to think in terms of healing and process rather than political expediency and profit. We need to be sensitive to this problem and empathize with those unfortunate people who are caught up in an extremely difficult situation.

Marijuana

Marijuana is the herb of the Aquarian age—it generally makes people feel good. Marijuana is a weed which grows ubiquitously. A weed is considered undesirable. Used responsibly we are able to alter our own consciousness or perception of the world and experience and feel things and people in a totally new way.

Marijuana, as a relaxant and a subtle mood elevator, has medical potentials which are enormous. What inhibits us is that the orthodox medical model classifies herbs or natural substances as "other"—outside the acceptable armamentarium; it does not recognize or want to recognize the inherent worth or value of such substances. The fact that this herb has been used for thousands of years for a vast array of medical ailments by cultures who are able to recognize that dis-ease and limited or imperfect perception are one and the same has failed to impress the medical "authorities."

Awareness and keen perception is directly related to the ability to concentrate, to pay attention to the immediate vision, to be in the *now*. As the energy level increases, the greater becomes the ability to see the immediate reality clearly. We become more aware of feelings, perceptions and movements which at a different level were not perceived and we were therefore unconscious of their reality. We may directly experience the universe in movement and in flow and realize that we are part of this movement. We allow ourselves to be opened up to a greater amount of energy—we become aware that we are receivers and transmitters of energy at various, continually changing levels of feelings, moods, and perceptions.

The change occurs when we recognize our addictions and impulses and consciously decide to act through conscious will; we control our emotional nature rather than having our emotional nature control us. We move from the gut level to that of the heart level where we feel and give out the harmonizing energy *love*. The revelation and the feelings of love result from the awareness and understanding that all things are essentially spiritual in nature regardless of their physical appearance. It is being able to see beyond the world of form that will gain us our freedom. We hear things differently, we see things more intensely, we get into the details of that with which we are interacting. Stifled awareness only clouds our vision and hence hides the aliveness and beauty of our own universe. It is for this reason that marijuana is gaining widespread acceptance though illicit. It has the ability to make us realize that there is a significance, direction, and purpose to our existence.

The dangers of marijuana are in the changing of the level and perception of reality and hence our intimate belief system. When used introspectively, it has the ability of letting you see and examine past actions from a space or level which is "higher" than that from which you normally have come. It is in this way also that marijuana can induce paranoia or anxiety; this new awareness may threaten the ego and the ego tries to defend itself or ward off impulses, ideas, or feelings which are greater than itself. This can be a painful, powerful struggle. However, if we understand that there is nothing to be lost and everything to be gained then perhaps we will view the experience with less trepidation and resistance. This movement from darkness into light is initiated by the self through subconsciousness and experienced consciously as new feelings, thoughts, emotions, and attitudes.

LSD-25, mescaline, psilocybin all act in a similar and more powerful fashion. Thus, one may perceive more intensely the vibrations of the universe be they colors, light, or sound which impinge upon our consciousness and are experienced as feelings. The more open or receptive you are, the higher the energy level, the more perceptive, the more sensitive, the more feeling you become.

The practical uses of marijuana for medical purposes are vast. Marijuana is a relaxant, however, like any other external agent, its individual effects are unpreditable. For some people it induces sleep, for others paranoid feelings, listlessness, apathy, the range of emotions are innumerable. However, the widespread use and self-medication of marijuana is an indication of its successfully fulfilling the need of people to relieve anxieties and tensions. Its pleasurable effects are mediated through its ability to relax mind and body. Marijuana would be an effective agent for the treatment of hypertension, peptic ulcer disease, ulcerative colitis, glaucoma, nausea and vomiting, muscular spasm, low back pain, asthma, angina; it is effective for any disease entity which has its causation in excess anxiety.

When we look at the therapeutic failures of the above dis-ease entities and compare them with the known effects of marijuana, we are led to the natural question: Why isn't this herb used for medicinal purposes?

The answer is painful because it strikes at the heart of two belief systems which appear to be diametrically opposed to each other. Psychosomatic medicine or wholistic medicine is just beginning to take hold and gain recognition of its viability. The problem it faces is that medicine has been developed along the lines of specialities and sub- specialties which create the myopic, tunnel vision of so much of the medicine being practiced today. To suggest that marijuana may have important therapeutic potentials would create a furor in most medical circles. The hypocrisy is somewhat overwhelming as we in the medical profession continue to prescribe drugs of doubtful efficacy for a wide range of idiopathic disorders whose results almost always are negligible.

As we "advance" to "higher" states of awareness and consciousness we may begin to use marijuana as a useful working tool to help open ourselves to the more subtle energies which emanate from within and without.

This herb has the ability to move one out of normal waking consciousness. As William James stated, normal waking consciousness "is but one type of consciousness, while all about it, parted from it by the filmiest of screens, there lie potential forms of consciousness entirely different. We may go through life without suspecting their existence; but apply the requisite stimulus, and at a touch they are there in all their completeness, definite types of mentality which probably somewhere have their field of application and adaptation. No account of the universe in its totality can be final which leaves these forms of consciousness disregarded."

Most people who use marijuana do not take the experience "seriously"; a separation is created and the herb is used as a diversion or recreational medium. Sometimes, inadvertently we present experiences to our conscious awareness that cannot be denied in terms of immediate and long-lasting relevance. The seeker consciously begins to realize that the life within presents an infinite variety of experiences and possibilities. He may begin to perceive the world as a series of movement, ever new, ever changing—a collage of images and impressions passing in front of his eyes. This opening up is the beginning of *real* health, a continuous flow of good feelings. The feelings emanate from within and are projected out into the world as a positive force or vibration.

The potential uses of strong marijuana used in conjunction with a guide or therapist who has worked through the emotional reactive process can provide the person with invaluable feedback regarding his own dynamic process and also give insight into where he is in his evolution.

LSD-25 works in a similar though more pronounced fashion than marijuana. Its power lies in its ability to induce the meditative state, to focus and concentrate the higher energies into conscious awareness. It is far less subtle than marijuana and we quickly learn how our emotions and feelings control us. We are immediately put into communication with our strongest desires, fears and wishes—the range of experience depends upon the state of where the person is at in his own evolution at that particular moment. He may focus his concentration to the objective outer reality or may focus his attention inward and perceive the infinite world of the mind. He may enter through this world into superconsciousness whereby the experiencer and the experience merge into a unity of ecstatic bliss whereupon the concept of self or personality "dissolves" and on examination after the experience he may understand that contact has been established with his essence. The doors of perception have been opened and the understanding of reality has been permanently changed.

The concept of using LSD-25 to heal oneself is based upon false premises. The concept that the subconscious mind is a repository of latent repressed drives and emotions which need to be examined consciously and dealt with creates the concept that we are somehow or other "sick" or imbalanced. This notion stems basically from Freudian psychology. If only we could find out and examine those aspects of ourselves which are creating pain and turmoil, then certainly we will experience health and well-being. The truth of the matter is that the subconscious is not only a repository and memory bank of one's personal experience in this life, but a memory bank which contains the entire history of man. All events are recorded and it is a sheer impossibility to root out those experiences which "objectively" are viewed as negative. All events are essentially neutral and it is only our interpretation of such happenings which color them positive or negative. It is futile to try to root out what we think are negative experiences, therefore it is really obligatory for us to move forward, learning from the past, and see life as an ever-expanding adventure in consciousness.

We cannot forcibly recreate our own rebirth. Regeneration and rebirth is the natural order of life and to try to enforce our own personal definition on how life should be and how it should be ordered is really tampering with the infinite power of the universe. Thus, while LSD-25 may provide vivid experiences into deeper aspects of being it should not be used as a tool to speed up the evolutionary process. This process is inherent within our own genetic coding. As we learn to understand the structure of the mind and its triad of self-consciousness, subconsciousness and underlying superconsciousness then we will be more respectful and accepting of how things are, realizing that in spite of all appearances, the universe is in a state of dynamic equilibrium and perfection—we share and partake of this perfection. To tamper, to manipulate, or forcibly impose our own personal will upon the primal Will is to invite disaster. Therein is the real danger of indiscriminant use of LSD-25.

LSD-25 used in a responsible, mature manner provides the healing profession an invaluable tool in helping people gain real insight into an aspect of reality which has been closeb tohthem. The use of this catalyst has been abused because it initially was not understood. The judicious use of mind-expanding drugs may alleviate the fear of death and its

attendant anxieties; break down destructive self-images; help
people to realize the infinite potential residing within themselves; give concrete evidence as to how their attitudes,
beliefs, and emotions help form reality and thereby lays the
groundwork for positive change.

The healing professions should move forward with caution,
humility, and *courage* and use all available tools particularly
those which can alleviate subjective existential suffering. As
long as we see each other as "sick" or as persons who need to
be controlled and are unable to recognize that there does indeed exist something greater than what appears before us,
then we are doomed to continue with a form of medicine that
is essentially nonprogressive and based on illusion. We use
the power of the intellectual mind and the ego to create
boundaries and perceptions of reality which appear so real
yet are only as real as the dreams we entertain each night.
We must look at our failures and seek alternatives. High
doses of thorazine, lithium, mood elevators, amphetamines,
steroids, antineoplastic agents, or broad-spectrum antibiotics
are but gross attempts to change behavior or alleviate symptomatic suffering which is time prove themselves to be of
marginal value, worthless or downright dangerous. We have
to put an end to this relentless poisoning and look for more
gentle healing agents.

   Just as there are the synthetic chemicals, which to date
number over 5,400, so are there herbal or natural substances
which are time-tested and very effective.

   We as a society have chosen collectively to continue taking chemical substances, even now admitting to ourselves
that these drugs create physiologic imbalances. Technology
has become our master not our servant. Just as we poison the
environment so have we chosen to poison ourselves. *Health* is
something to be worked for, to be attained, a struggle. It

means changing; it does not come in the form of a pill. It's time we stopped fooling ourselves.

Mechanistic medicine will continue on its own path until it is recognized within and without the medical community that a change in philosophy and approach is needed—this change will be commensurate with the desire of the people to change themselves and embrace health.

Change is often difficult but once we see life as a process with no beginning and no end then we have taken a tremendous step in relieving ourselves of responsibility for other people's dilemmas. This does not rule out understanding and compassion. Our "problem" is that we are not collectively consciously evolved to that point of seeing the divinity within each and every one of us, particularly within ourselves. Man is afraid to identify himself with spirit and to affirm his own greatness. Sooner or later we will all do this in our own way and in our own time.

The whole concept of mental illness, appropriate behavior, and correct perception of reality are seriously being contested today as we begin to understand at various levels that we all see *it* differently and that because of the profoundness and challenges of life we attempt to build a structure of beliefs to try to explain reality to ourselves.

The structure and belief systems stay intact until one either undergoes a spontaneous change or growth which is the natural order of the universe or makes a conscious decision through the pain of awareness that there is more to *it* than we are led to believe; the material objective world is but one reality.

7

Death and Dying

Liberation and freedom in their deepest sense relate to the internalization and conscious realization of our own immortality.

All manifestation which finds expression in the universe is derived from the one source and we are intimately related and supported by this life power. It is as if the Creator had divided itself into an infinite number of beings and manifestations so that it could experience itself through these expressions. However, we do not identify ourselves with the power of the universe which moves of its own accord—that is to say it is totally free. Each man intuitively strives for freedom and this freedom goes beyond the freedom of choice or expression—this freedom is derived from knowing, realizing that one is part of and not apart from the creative intelligence which we call *God*.

It is because we do not relate to nature as part of ourselves that we feel fear, isolation, and loneliness. There is no separation. The world is a metaphor with an incredible array of beings at various stages of evolvement. Many of us have not embraced or recognized that which we are; it is not that we have to become something we already are, but we are not consciously aware that we are and this creates the illusion of existential or nihilistic loneliness.

Perhaps the most difficult thing to comprehend is to reconcile the negative aspects which manifest in the world today. The world is moving through its own evolutionary process just as each individual is moving through his own unique guided unfoldment. The tension which drives the universe and generates the desire for creativity appears within all things. As we unfold we may see and conciously realize our entire lives as dramas that reflect our inherent beauty and perfection—not only of ourselves but of all creation. It is at this point that we may realize the illusion of time, the realization that there is no beginning, that there is no end, that the cosmos is a life force which is unceasingly working, through us, toward its own liberation.

The devil or Satan is that aspect of ourselves which creates separation or illusion and keeps most of us on an endless treadmill of desires and addictions that blind us to reality. We are at a point in evolution where we still are in darkness; most people are suffering from a spiritual malaise, however, this desire to reach out and experience our higher selves is spreading. Our lives may be seen as an "upward" expansion to self-realization through the process of time. Those beings who act out from limited belief systems continue to do so until their consciousness changes to that level where they are dissatisfied—this dissatisfaction is a result of stasis, dis-ease, and boredom which runs counter to the creative impulse and rhythm of the universe. Our dis-eases are overt messages which are letting us know that we must learn to attune ourselves to the higher energies—that is to say recognize and reach out for spiritual awareness.

It is for this reason that one's attitudes, beliefs and emotional reaction intimately affect our health on a day-to-day basis. It is also for this reason that change is not only necessary but life-giving. The word *change* implies the breaking down of old structured habits or thinking processes. Change is the inherent law of the universe which continuously creates as it destroys. It is important to realize that this destruction or death is a renewal or purification process because it gives birth to that which is new and alive. Thus, through personal evolution we die to our old selves, giving up outdated or limited belief systems. This takes courage, acceptance, and the spirit of adventure, however, the driving force and encouragement to do this is self-impelling and is felt within all things which live.

The word death not only implies physical death but psychological death as well. Simply stated, death is the cessation of the heart beat or pulsatile force where there is a departure of the spirit from body consciousness. It is an axiom of most all philosophies that inherent upon death is rebirth; as proof one only need to witness this redundant theme in nature: Spring always follows winter; a continuous never-ending cycle of creation—death—rebirth. Just as nature undergoes death and renewal so do we in a very real way. The body undergoes total cellular regeneration every two years or so: there is a continuous exchange of assimilation and elimination, anabolism and catabolism.

All things are created out of energy in a particular form which gives it a unique identity; as all things are reflections of energy one may deduce the immortality of all things—"energy can neither be created or destroyed, only transformed."

It is our resistance to change which creates turmoil, havoc and dis-ease. This resistance creates opposition to the forces within ourselves which are continuously impelling us to move, experience, and create. We can only resist the inexorable flow and rhythms for so long, this is the eternal struggle of the higher self and the lower-self (ego) which must in time submit to the higher energies. The beauty of it all is that we have everything to gain and nothing to lose except illusion and suffering. This giving up of your old image is psychologically a death experience because the old tapes in programming (habits) are engrained within the matrix of your personality and tend to control your action. It is the concept of acting from either *my will* or *thy will.* When Jesus ordered his ego, "Satan, get thee behind me," he was referring to his internal struggle to let go of his lower self and embrace his spiritual self which he knew must manifest itself.

While there is much interest and intellectualization today in this country about reincarnation, out-of-body experiences, telepathy, clairvoyance, astrology, mediumship, and psychic phenomena there has been little advancement in the more humane treatment of those individuals who are undergoing the death process. *The Tibetan Book of the Dead* is a holy book which has arrived in the West to help enlighten Western man and expand his consciousness. This book not only acknowledges immortality as an acknowledged undebatable fact but explains in detail the death process and the importance of the person's state of mind at the moment of death. This is an area of medicine which has been sorely avoided because it deals with our most profound and deepest anxieties. We accept this reality of death for the present and realize fully that any change in our approach and attitudes toward dying people will not change until there is a demand for it. As long as medical schools do not deal with reality, and see life as a linear process progressing from point "A" to point "B" then we will continue to see the resultant abuses and false heroics which are daily occurrences in our intensive care units and hospital wards.

Before one "passes on" or "passes away" the body's breathing pattern changes, this is clinically called *Cheynne-Stokes respiration* and is a cardinal sign of impending death. The body is preparing the consciousness for the shock of

death—this is extremely merciful and helpful in those individuals who identify with their bodies or egos. However, in
the death throes, a carbon dioxide narcosis is induced which
creates a separateness or disassociation from ordinary reality
(this is often described as a euphoria), there are hallucinations. Patients on the chronic respiratory wards suffering
from emphysema and bronchitis continually move in and out
of altered states of consciousness—these hallucinations are
but different realities and are termed hallucinations only
because they have not been consciously experienced before,
hence the reason for psychotic reactions in individuals who
suddenly open up into the subconscious and consciously
become aware of material which previously was hidden.

As the body mercifully prepares us for a gradual
withdrawal under a self-induced trance state doctors are
desperately trying to save the patient when in reality the outcome for survival or death is beyond our power. I am not advocating that no attempts be made by the physician to
"save" the patient, what I am advocating is a sane approach
to the terminal patient where our *attitude* should be toward
support and comfort—it is vitally important that the *mind* be
put to rest because our immediate beliefs, fears and anxieties
are self-realized before us!! It is not unlike an LSD-25 experience where we may experience negative emotions and fears
which are but projections of our ego.

An example of the tampering process can be well illus-
trated by the following situation:

An elderly man had metastatic bone disease secondary to
a primary adenocarcinoma of the lung. He was also suffering
from pneumonia and congestive heart failure. By all esti-
mates this man was certainly dying. His main medical problem was the relief of his bone pain which created severe continuous agony. The man was kept on an artificial ventilator
because of the respiratory failure, a condition where he was
not able to bring enough oxygen into his lungs to support his

life. When an insufficient supply of oxygen was not available he suffered from hypoxia which affected the entire metabolism of his body; along with this problem was the problem of carbon dioxide buildup which resulted from a decreased ability of the lungs to eliminate this potential toxin. Thus there was a reversal of the blood gases whereby the oxygen content of the body was decreased and the carbon dioxide was increased, leading to a clinical condition known as *carbon oxide narcosis*. In situations where there was no artificial ventilation the man would have slipped into a coma and mercifully died not suffering any pain. It is at this point due to a combination of social, moral, and legal responsibilities that a physician will play heroics and tamper with an incredibly benevolent system which ensures the quiet peaceful demise of the patient.

The decision was made and the patient was hooked up to a respirator which forcibly drove air into the man's lungs and decreased the carbon dioxide. This reversal and normalization of the blood gases aroused the patient to waking consciousness. Upon being conscious the patient cried out in pain because he was now tuned into his body racked with metastatic bone disease—this is a gruesome pain resulting from a tumor pushing out against the periosteum of the bone. His pain was recognized and he was immediately given morphine—we were very careful not to give him too much because we were aware of the effect of morphine upon the respiratory system (morphine has a depressant effect upon the physiology of respiration). The drug altered the man's rate of respiration, however, he was on a respirator and we saw the interesting situation where the man was fighting the machine—his body's respiratory rate influenced by the drug effect and working against a standard set rate imposed by the mechanical respirator. The man's bone pain disappeared as his consciousness was altered by the drug effect and by the alteration once again of the blood gases. A sample was taken of this man's blood to see the state of his blood gases which characteristically showed a decreased oxygen and elevated carbon dioxide—the man had lapsed back into carbon dioxide narcosis. The machine was stepped up once again to correct this potential life threatening situation and equilibrated to normal or as close to normal as possible—that is to say high oxygen low carbon dioxide. This created a change in consciousness and moved the patient out of his coma as there was increased oxygen supply to the brain—the man becomes conscious again of his pain and the cycle continued until the man died of exhaustion.

A decision could have been made to turn off the respirator. It is much more difficult to turn off a respirator than it is to turn one on. We get caught in a difficult situation because we are not seeing the inevitable process and are trying to save a life which is well beyond saving. This patient was subjected to mental and physical torture as he repeatedly moved in and out of coma where he was able to contemplate and experience his approaching demise. He was also subject to innumerable procedures necessary to monitor the blood gases. The method is simple—one simply sticks a needle into the femoral or radial artery, withdraws the blood and measures its oxygen and carbon dioxide saturations. We rapidly lose sight that we are stabbing and inflicting pain into a live human being; this is overlooked as we battle and try to maintain a clinically suitable level of acid-base physiology.

Not only is the patient subject to various bodily insults to keep tabs of the situation but the environment of most intensive care units is such as to *not* promote the well-being of the gravely ill patient. The lights are harsh and are kept on continuously. The patient is continuously being badgered because of compulsive orders to have this or that procedure done far too frequently. The fear of litigation is continuously influencing the decisions of a medical team when they manage the patient. The wise, humane course of action is often not taken because society and a good lawyer can easily convince a jury of errors of omission.

What generally happens is that a certain point is passed and the team commits itself to a certain course of standardized treatment, generally one which will employ the "greatest" advances in technology to support the life forces. This is valuable and real when the condition of the patient is such that there are reasonable expectations that recovery will occur, remembering always that gentleness, rest, good nutrition, and silence will in itself help the healing process far more than a cursory examination in a crowded ward, staffed by exhausted, anxious doctors who are unable to continuously deal with such crisis situations.

We often find ourselves treating one iatrogenic disaster after another as we crudely, empirically try to reestablish a sense of equilibrium. We are not fully conscious of the fact that very sick people do not have the strength or resistance to be abused and assaulted with various invasive techniques and unphysiological doses of drugs which are marginal at best as we attempt to prolong the life of the patient. The medical team often has to consider the onus of litigation as it is being compelled to treat a person regardless of the merits of the treatment—a "good" lawyer can prove that not enough was done. It is an extremely sensitive situation. Sometimes doing nothing is doing something—just as sometimes doing something does something. It is the nature and quality of that something which the medical profession has to take a good hard look at! We often commit ourselves to a course of disaster that works against the best interests of the patient.

The stress, pain, and cost which is inflicted is often enormous and very often we effect a cure only to see a relapse in a day, week or month. The attitudes and feelings of the patient rarely come into the picture. Rational, mechanistic science knows best or so we are led to believe. A sense of humor is always necessary for even on the gallows the condemned man may still retain his sense of humor. When it is decided that the patient is not going to make it, the chaplain, priest, rabbi or whoever is summoned and a certain ritual is performed. We can only imagine the thoughts of a patient who in his stuporous condition perceives the form of a religious man performing some sort of liturgy upon his body. It's OK if you're prepared for it, but if you're not . . . think about it—there is no fear if you believe in continuous life, but if your belief system sees itself as a linear process of "A to B," beginning and end, you can easily project the feelings of fear, terror, regret or whatever as you silently try to make some sense of your rapidly ending life.

Today's hospitals are totally inadequate in serving the needs of dying people. It is an area of little concern and great insensitivity because the human being defends and closes off to that which is so personal and so threatening. Every time we confront another's death we must confront our own. This is extremely painful if our beliefs do not include a certain degree of optimism. There are those who state that these belief systems were designed strictly for the reason of allowing the person a less turbulent passage. Should that be true— that is to say, life is but a brief moment in time—then there really is no harm in deluding yourself is there? However, if we see the universe as essentially merciful and benevolent, and our beliefs have a definite bearing as to how we react to life after death, then we can infer that we are way off course in administering humane, compassionate dispensation.

What are the alternatives?

There are many and one must focus upon creating a positive, harmonious, tranquil feeling within the environment of gravely ill patients. Soft lights, warm colors, beautiful music, a positive attitude of support and love from the staff is what is needed in easing the burden of death. In many cultures dying is seen as a time of celebration, not of mourning. The more "primitive" cultures are more attuned to reality; they recognize the endless process of life and see death not only as a change but as liberation. To some this may sound as fantasy—is it any more or less fantastic than what is going on today in our modern hospitals? One system believes in heroics and battling the forces of nature while the other recognizes the limitations of our ability to cure others and offers in its stead sensitivity, kindness, and humaneness.

If we look very closely and witness the death process we may see some extraordinary positive events occur regarding the experience of liberation on death. For example, I witnessed two moribund patients who upon their death had erections and ejaculated—an embarrassment to those attending but its symbolic import cannot be dismissed. This final release has been described by numerous patients who have been revived as an ecstatic, exhilarating experience and many who have undergone this experience no longer fear death because they had recognized and experienced the "Grand Illusion."

The other attitude which needs to be collectively understood is that the doctors are not responsible for a person's *demise*. All physicians operate from what they believe to be correct and it's only their egos which want to take credit for saving a life, it is also the ego which creates the pain and suffering when a patient dies.

Of course there are variations in between where mistakes are made which have created physiological disasters—most often however these are errors of *commission* rather than *omission*—"Do no harm" is still the cardinal rule of medicine. We still suffer from the Ben Casey/Dr. Kildare syndrome.

The British have a very humanistic approach regarding terminal or dying people. They have built, in London, a hospital solely designed for the supportive care of dying cancer patients—there is no heroic measures, unnecessary surgery; no use of chemotherapy—there is an acceptance here that death is very much a part of life. Also, the British use a tonic called Brompton's mixture which is a combination of heroin (morphine), cocaine, and gin. People are eased into their deaths feeling no pain, only pleasure.

The new age medicine may even be a bit more venturesome and send the patient off with a real high abolishing the illusion of death before the departure by the responsible use of LSD or psilocybin. There are no doubt individuals who are so moralistically rigid that they would react to such treatment as wrong and grievously misguided while they live the lie of quiet desperation and fear never knowing what it really means to feel and experience the inner self. Interestingly enough we see throughout history the use of hallucinogens and opiates found in nature to help man in his journey of self-discovery. The English writer Aldous Huxley, noted that all naturally occurring sedatives, narcotics, euphorics and hallucinogens were discovered by man before the dawn of civilization by simple experimentation. Huxley himself was given LSD just before he died. Unfortunately we cannot get his own report as to how it went, however, Laura Huxley, in *This Timeless Moment*, tells us "the ceasing of life was not a drama at all, but like a piece of music just finishing so gently."

The pioneering work in this area is currently being done at the Maryland Psychiatric Hospital where LSD-25 is given to patients who are suffering from terminal cancer. This modality is used to help these people work through the fear of death. The potentials are enormous, we need only be honest about our real needs and fears and take necessary steps to assuage them.

I envision the day when this society decides to create facilities where humanistic medicine may be practiced unfettered by the oppressive forces of orthodox hospital medicine and an individual will be allowed to die graciously, painlessly, and supportively. This would be the actualizing of knowledge into wisdom and confirm our humaneness to each other; it only takes the courage of our beliefs to actualize such a situation. We are all free agents; whether we are consciously aware of this or not is basically a matter of our own personal evolution, however, we must recognize and insist that each person has the inherent right to die consciously and, hopefully, in a state of grace.

8

Hospitals Today, Healing Centers Tomorrow

Today's hospitals reflect a system of thought and a particular belief system. Modern hospital medicine today is based upon an orthodox medical model which is materialistic, mechanistic, superficial, exorbitantly expensive, and totally nonindividualized. Besides being locked into a particular way of practicing medicine, the physical environment in which we place sick people often works against the best interests of the patient. There are six essential elements contributing to physical and mental health:

sunlight
fresh air
sound nutrition
exercise
clean water
hope

The degree to which we do not provide ourselves with these basic essentials is the degree to which we jeopardize our health.

Today's hospitals are environmentally unsound. Not only are they breeding grounds for a host of pathogenic and increasingly resistant strains of bacteria, but they also are reservoirs of foul air, poor quality food, a hectic noisy environment, a "sterile" environment run by bureaucrats whose major interest is in the economic viability of the institution. When a hospital's viability is totally dependent upon the amount of surgery that must be done to keep it in the black then you can perhaps project the motivation of those people who perform the surgery. When a doctor has spent a good many years learning surgical technique it is obvious that his personal survival is dependent on the amount of surgery he must do. Unconsciously or consciously this creates a tremendous pressure to operate in many cases where a conservative approach would do as well. To illustrate the point, it is routine to take out a child's tonsils and adenoids, the major justification being that these are unnecessary organs within the body. Everything in the body has its place and function. Just because medical science says that it is functionless does not mean that this is true.

We must remember that medical science is in its infancy and the laws of healing are not fully understood. The laws of healing, both mental and physical, involve the following principles:

1. The subconscious mind controls and regulates moment to moment all the vital processes within the organism, below the level of conscious awareness.

2. The subconscious mind is always amenable to suggestion. The law of suggestion is the mode in which one affects, positively or negatively, the subconscious processes. You can literally talk yourself into a diseased state just as you may talk yourself out of it.

3. The subconscious mind works through a process of deductive reasoning; it has no ability to discriminate or analyze incoming suggestions. It accepts as true whatever impressions are given it, visual or auditory. The advertising in-

dustry and political propagandists use the law of suggestion continuously.

4. Healing works through the agency of subconsciousness to effect positive states of mind and body. As Carl Jung stated, we are all linked together via a "collective subconscious." It is through this agency that we may receive healing influences from the unseen or spiritual aspect of oneself. "Ask and you will receive."

It is through understanding the structure of our mind that we may begin to understand the phenomenon of faith healing, healing at a distance, telepathic communication, the positive effects of the ritualistic, scientific use of sound and color in healing, and the power of prayer. We need to understand the relationship of the self-conscious to the subconsious, to the superconscious, realizing that they are different aspects of the same thing. Through a process of education and learning we may begin to consciously suggest positive ideas and images to the subconscious which over a process of time will recreate healthy states of mind and body. This is the basis of the yoga philosophy which allows the practitioner to gain control over his emotions and, through self-discipline, learn the art of relaxation which is the key to a balanced autonomic nervous system. We may learn this technique as well. The process of self-hypnosis or progressive relaxation will in time, once the art of suggestion and the correct language of subconsciousness is learned, also create positive states of mind and body.

A person who is in emotional turmoil needs an environment that is both supportive and aesthetically pleasing. New age crisis centers will be developed that understand these needs. All efforts will be directed toward creating an atmosphere of tranquility. The judicious use of water therapy, massage, and sauna, to help induce bodily relaxation will be employed. Once a person feels safe in such a situation then meaningful communication may occur and the underlying problems may be brought to conscious awareness. The person will be allowed to express whatever feelings necessary for them, without the fear of being institutionalized or labeled. The emphasis will continually be based on process and education. Compassion, reassurance and individual responsibility will be the basis of new age crisis centers and healing centers in general. We must move to an understanding of the laws of healing and embrace them and incorporate them in our day to day life. Nature is the greatest healer there is; use of nature—the sun, the fresh air, and the soothing green—will enhance and speed the healing process.

Hypnosis and self-hypnosis is an extremely powerful tool for healing and for prevention. It works directly with the laws of suggestion which are the basis of health and happiness. There is much confusion and misunderstanding of this tool. It is very simple once learned and has far-reaching consequences for the individual who uses it consistently. Basically, hypnosis is a state of increased receptivity where the subconscious mind is in the foreground and you may communicate directly with it, remembering that the subconscious is always amenable to suggestion. The rational, intellectual, self-conscious mind is put to rest and you gain direct access to the machinery of the body. The art of self-hypnosis lies in the ability to put yourself into this subjective, receptive state, and then through correct formulation of suggestions impress on the subconscious whatever it is you desire.

As long as our hospitals are run by bureaucrats and analogous to a factory mass production system using such techniques as chemicals or unnecessary surgery, we will continue to see the iatrogenic disasters which are the root of the malpractice crisis. Our nearsightedness, our overreliance on technology, our insensitive disregard for the sanctity and inherent healing potentials within the body all create forces and factors working against the recovery of the sick person.

Our stubborn commitment to medical dogma which deals mainly with pathology and the refusal by those in power who control and direct research and funding to allow new ideas based on more universal concepts to be allowed to be explored and researched, create the stifling negative attitude which affect all of us.

There is a trememdous ego investment in being the one who discovers the latest cure for this or that disease entity; the medical profession is suffering from the sin of hubris, an arrogance that keeps it from seeing the collapse of a system not working within the commonsense fundamental laws which govern healing. We are all caught up in it in varying degrees and are being tyrannized by a system of thought which is not producing the cures it claims it makes. We are great at identifying and describing pathology; we love to categorize and classify, but when it comes down to safe, effective inexpensive treatment we are solidly lacking. The reason for this is obvious: There is a tremendous lack of imagination and courage within the medical community. The creative process which is essential for life is stifled and generally buried in medical school. The medical student's entire time is spent memorizing endless facts from endless books, regurgitating irrelevant data, living under the illusion that the accumulation of knowledge produces a sensitive, thinking human being—a doctor. New ideas are shunned and historically anyone who rebels or questions the prevailing dogma is either quietly ostracized or labeled defective in some manner or other. The medical-school rebel pays a heavy price for freedom and most young doctors are too afraid to speak out against their "fathers," yet if we are to be of real service to ourselves and to the community we must recognize that reason without love creates death and stagnation.

We are now faced with a new phenomenon—the young coming to maturity questioning the old and creating something new, vibrant, and alive. It is not that the elders have nothing to offer us because obviously there are many wise, concerned professionals with vast and deep experiences to share with us. The problem is a lack of dialogue or communication and a denial of basic human values and needs. We as doctors cannot really do the job effectively if we ourselves are troubled, upset, and confused. If we see man as essentially defective we will create a system which will perpetuate that belief. If we see man as an evolving being whose growth is dependent upon compassion and understanding then we are committed to changing our institutions from hospitals to healing centers so we may foster growth and health.

Virtually any doctor who has had extensive experience will relate the truth that virtually all disease is really a mind/body phenomenon. (This of course excludes physical trauma where modern medicine and technology is quite advanced and life saving.) We have to grasp the concept of universalism, to see that the uplifting of an individual enhances and enriches the collective experience of the society. The only real role society has is a commitment to concern itself with peace, love, freedom, and happiness. The degree to which we can integrate these precepts into our daily lives will determine the degree to which we will experience the ideals.

The consciousness of society is expanding rapidly through the miracle of mass media and instant communication. We are becoming increasingly aware that the internal dynamics and relative health or disease of each individual has a profound effect upon the well-being of the whole society. The degree to which we acknowledge this awareness consciously is the degree to which we will collectively commit ourselves to building a new world order based upon what we truly want, not what we think we want. If we are able to see life as an expansive creative force always working towards its own liberation, then perhaps we can respond by developing, through insight, intelligence and imagination, an educational system which addresses itself to the questions of health and a medical system that will allow itself to expand and in-corporate new ideas. We need various approaches to healing, but we need to see that the methods applied are safe, gentle, compassionate, and inexpensive.

We need to return to fundamental, commonsense princi-pals. Rest and mental relaxation is absolutely essential before the healing process can occur. The human touch, compas-sion, and understanding supplies the real magic in the heal-ing process. Just as each cell in the body is dependent upon the consciousness of the individual, society is dependent upon the collective consciousness of people. If our values and pri-orities and life's energies are misdirected then we pay the price in terms of disease and ill-health. Everything effects everything else.

The coronary care unit is an interesting phenomenon. A young man of 35 experiences severe retrosternal chest pain radiating to his left arm, he also notes sweating, anxiety, pain in the jaw, perhaps epigastric discomfort. He knows enough—having watched endless medical dramas on TV—that he may be having a "heart attack." Just this occurrence and its recognition increases his heart rate and further com-promises the heart's functioning; an alert goes out, the sirens scream, the man is hustled into an ambulance, the anxiety and state of tension is reflected not only in the patient, as his mind races trying to answer and rectify the implications of this happening, but in the attendants as well who are well aware that time is critical—this man needs hospital care as soon as possible.

If the man survives the dash to the hospital without suf-fering a fatal arrhythmia he is rushed to the coronary care unit where he is hooked up to a monitor where his heart rate and rhythm are carefully observed. His blood pressure and his pulse are carefully watched. Repeated EKGs are taken to see if characteristic acute changes have taken place. Blood is taken to see if there is a rise of certain enzymes which indi-cate cell damage. A team of cardiologists listen, observe, and try to make a diagnosis. Various drugs are on hand to control blood pressure and arrhythmias.

What is understood but not taken into account is the psychological impact of this scene. The patient is continuously aware that his heart, his life pulsatile force, is capable at any moment of failing and thereby end his life. An eventuality that most people have not really thought about particularly at a young age. That this possibility is *real*, that death may happen at any time, can in itself create tremendous panic and anxiety. The patient is isolated, left alone in a dark quiet room where the only sound is the monitoring and steady beat of his own heart. For many people this is an excruciatingly painful process. Generally, psychological factors are ignored, the person is left alone to cope with this situation as well as possible.

What is particularly distressing is the realization that the implementation of coronary care units throughout the United States has had virtually no real effect on lowering the mortality rate for victims of acute myocardial infarctions.

We must be doing something wrong! The expense and effort have not measureably improved one's chance of survival. This is understandable if one examines the situation from a distance. We rush a victim from his natural, familiar, comfortable environment, to a sterile, imposing environment where he is denied access to support from those whom he especially needs, particularly if he believes he is going to die. We are not seeing the patient, we are not recognizing the agony, the regrets, the desire for communication a person may have at this crucial point of his life. The machines take over, a clinical detachment pervades the CCU. The patient is but another grim statistic lending further evidence to the epidemic of early death due to cardiac exhaustion. We are not seeing the human being any more—we only see a body, a heart which needs to be chemically controlled.

It is an interesting phenomenon, reported by a cardiologist who has extensive experience that approximately 30 percent of patients with chronic heart disease will intimate a strong intuition as to when they will die. The will to live, the will to die resides within the person. Modern technology, no matter how sophisticated will not override those psychological impulses which create the physical reality of life or death.

We continuously work against ourselves—the frenetic pace, the sense of panic, the nonacceptance of letting life be, the inherent fear among many physicians to acknowledge that they really are not in control of what is happening before them. The need to do something which often is not dictated by good clinical judgment but by fear that an "error" of omission will or could be used in a court of law for malpractice—the hysteria brought upon the physician by the relatives and families who have bought the lie of modern medicine's omnipotence.

All these subtle forces and factors contribute to the management and often abuse of the patient. Most of the time is spent dealing with technology, lab results, and such—where is the human support? The touching, the creation of a warm human atmosphere between human beings? It is often the small, "insignificant" actions which determine whether a patient lives or dies. One of the most profound experiences of my medical career happened in an intensive care unit. I could feel the need of the patient for human contact, I held this man's hand and he clasped it intuitively knowing that energy can pass from one person to another. My senior resident saw this action and criticized it as being histrionic and unprofessional—the laying on of hands is strictly *verboten*, superstitious nonsense, a relic of the past, science and technology have moved past such pleasantries. We pay an awful price for our insensitivities. What creates this callousness, aloofness, and insensitivity? This insensitivity is a product of cynicism; nonhumanistic medical schools; bitter egotistical professors who lay their trip of the school of hard knocks upon their students, endless data and research material which are ineffective and inconclusive; on-call schedules which create continuous anxiety and exhaustion on the would-be doctors. Endless schedules and conferences supplying a great deal of meaningless data, trying to prove the effectiveness of this or that therapy. The unbelievable bureaucracy and constant fear of being sued. The lure of material success; if you only hold on long enough and get your speciality then the struggle is over. Little or no time for personal development, a hectic schedule where personal needs are not met. The belief that the doctor still is lord and master; the refusal to abdicate some responsibility to the nursing staff and aides who spend most of the time with the patients and generally are more knowledgeable as to what is going on. The total separation of mind and body, the concept that the patient is a diseased organ system; the uptightness of the medical profession to review honestly its successes and its failures. The constant glorification of its successes; the quiet avoidance and denial of its ever-present "failures." The ignoring of the placebo effect in medicine which has been so beautifully documented in endless drug trials, the realization that healing is intimately related to the belief system of both the doctor and the patient. The abhorrence and fear of something new or different which is not scientifically proven, and yet so much of current therapy is not scientifically proven.

The continual use of jargon and terminology, while impressive sounding only belies the ignorance and non-understanding of innumerable disease processes. Many doctors have difficulty in communicating and seeing their patients as people; there is an overwhelming need for honesty, a need to admit that he does not really understand and thereby establish an honest working relationship with the patient. The medical student is isolated from the outside world; he is unable to see himself as part of a system which operates from a conceptual framework established in the late 1800s. There is the subtle imposition to deny creativity and to stifle within the student alternative conceptualizations of reality. And he is encouraged to faithfully repeat the latest gospel from this or that authority whose new method or therapy is in vogue (but will eventually fall out of favor when some new researcher takes a closer look at what is really happening). He is taught that knowledge and wisdom come from books and he only needs to memorize the incredible array of literature to become a competent doctor. Thinking for yourself is not highly recommended particularly if you want to get the right job.

We need to establish recycling centers where people can rest and learn techniques based on knowledge to regenerate their lives and hopefully allow their experience to be more meaningful. We have to let go of those attitudes and beliefs which are working against us and move toward actions which will enhance our well-being and make our experiences more enjoyable.

The new age healing centers will be implicitly holistic in approach operating from several philosophical bases. The responsibility for restoring people back to health is a process of integration of mind and body where the person who is sick will take an active part in trying to understand the basis of illness, and those who help support and nurture the patient back to health will share a joint responsibility. It will be a group effort operating from the premise that those energies which help to restore the patient to balance are universal energies and we as healers will work in communion with nature for the restoration of good health. The concept that we are all emerging sentient beings at various stages of evolution will be implicitly understood and the sacredness and sanctity of the body will be respected.

The healing community will *not* be based on *time* or money; the healing process is one of gradual reorientation, recognizing that disease can be a path to self-understanding and that one need not be punished financially or otherwise for suffering or being sick.

The stigma of labeling people in terms of this or that disease will be minimized, not because we are trying to deny reality, but because we are beginning to understand the tremendous power of suggestion and belief. Your concept and image of yourself is fundamental to what you project to the world. It is essentially how we think of ourselves and others which create the relative ease or dis-ease of our experience. Freudian psychology concentrates on that area of the personal subconscious where the negative conditioning and attitudes lie. The theory being that if insight is gained into innumerable conflicted ideas then you may gain increasing energy and freedom as your thought patterns are not so involved in self-conscious preoccupation. The problem here is that so much time is spent in the garbage can that in the same time you could direct your energies into building *new* conceptualizations of self. Our consciousness is unlimited and yet by the nature of how we see ourselves, we continuously limit our perspective and growth. As you begin to expand you can clearly see back into your past clearly and not suffer from guilt, shame, and recrimination. We need to see the present as a process built upon the past, but always to keep our sights forward. That same energy which is used to explore the past can be used just as effectively to recreate ourselves as something more alive and creative.

The new age healing centers will be diametrically opposed to what is going on in today's modern hospitals which are environmentally toxic, where the food is of poor quality, where the staff is overworked or bored, where the treatment is prepackaged and not individualized. The lack of fresh air, good lighting, and the lack of a warm, upbeat atmosphere will all be eliminated as we accept the set and setting as important for healing to take place as any other factor.

Light and its effect on our health is often ignored in the

therapeutic efforts of allopathic medicine. Until recently, the function of the pineal gland in human physiology was unknown and thought to represent a vestigal organ—like the thymus gland which was subsequently discovered to be intimately involved in determining and developing the immune system of the body.

The ancient Egyptians referred to the pineal gland as the "seat of the soul," the "third eye," or the "mind's eye." What is intimated here is a direct relationship between the third eye or pineal gland and the *conscious* light energy which is being transmitted to the earth moment to moment by the sun.

Scientifically, we now know that the pineal gland is a photoreactive organ which is directly connected to the pituitary gland via the hypothalamus. We also know scientifically that it is innervated by the superior cervical sympathetic ganglion of the autonomic nervous system. We also know scientifically that the pineal gland is intensely metabolically active as indicated by high levels of norepinepherine, serotonin, melatonin, histamine, acetlycholine, 5-methoxyindole, and 5-thdroxyindole acetic acids; these are all the *known* neurohumors of the brain which regulate and mediate the nervous activity of its 15 trillion individual cells.

Conscious evolution is the result of chemical change experienced within the body. The lifeforce, or Kundalini, within the body via the sympathetic nervous system activates the pineal gland and opens the mind's eye to interior vision. This in turn activates and balances the pituitary gland and brings about harmony. This is an evolutionary process.

Many of the ancient medical practitioners knew this intuitively. They understood the direct and immediate relationship between the conscious, living, healing, supporting rays of the sun and its effect upon all life. Our lives obviously are totally dependent upon this continuous, unconditional flow of energy. Light, the limitless light of the Qabalah, is the conscious, living energy which is both the creator and the sustainer of all things.

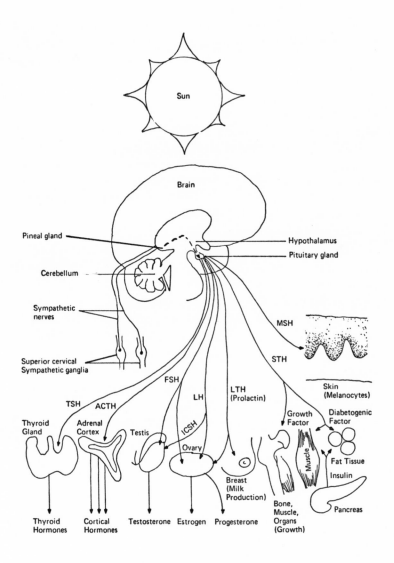

Science through spectroscopy has broken light down into its electromagnetic properties. When light is bent through a prism it reflects the seven colors of the visible spectrum, the colors of the rainbow, red, orange, yellow, green, blue, indigo, violet. This living light not only has physical visible properties but it has mathematical musical properties as well. These seven colors relate to the seven notes of the musical scale as well as to the seven glandular systems of the body as well as to the seven occult planets in astrology.

One only has to look at the word *Qabalah* and know its meaning and thereby learn the secret of healing. The Qabalah, the ancient wisdom, means receptivity. We need only become receptive to the light which is omnipresent and tune into the vibrations and music of the universe. This is the real secret of healing, the "healing" of the subconscious by the infinite power of the universal primal energy of the universe, God, which is always within us and always staring us right in the face. We only have to look at the sun and all of nature and reflect on what is behind it to realize the grandeur and infinite sea of consciousness which sustains us and the entire universe. Now that we understand this we need only to use our intelligence cooperatively and unconditionally to reap this boundless energy to help us individually and collectively.

Before technology came into being, and science "forgot" the subjective aspect of life, solariums were employed to heal the sick. We need to reconstruct in this society healing centers which use what is available and free to promote healing. The sun is the greatest healer there is and along with fresh air, good food, moderate exercise, and clean air we can re-educate ourselves and re-experience greater degrees of well-being. The only thing required is the permission from ourselves to partake of our natural inheritance. Within the simplicity of such an idea lies its profundity because we have just managed to make life so incredibly complicated!

Nature will heal us, if we allow it to and are receptive to its healing energies. The sun will not only heal our bodies and minds but will supply us with an unlimited, clean, ecologically perfect supply of energy, once we decide to commit ourselves to harnessing solar energy. The technology is there, all we need is the collective will to do it.

As the mind is able to relax, so will the body which will then become receptive to the universal healing energies (love) which are present at all times. Relaxation, happiness, humanness, and a sense of humor will be the operating characteristics for those who want to share in this important aspect of human endeavor. The precepts of "Do no harm" and "Physician, heal thyself" will be paramount within the consciousness of those people who will participate within the healing community.

Architecturally, the healing center will be aesthetic, warm, and pleasing to the human eye. The intelligent use of colors and tones will be consciously employed to enhance the healing milieu. All efforts will be made to help the individual attain peace of mind and teach that temporary discomfort is a potential growth experience.

As in any society there will be those people who will resist, reject, and scorn such centers because they are not scientific enough or because they threaten their belief system and desire to control. There will be regular hospitals which will still operate on a structured, money-making proposition, as long as they are needed. There will always be hospitals which are needed to deal with acute trauma or other surgical emergencies. These places will be there as long as there are enough people who want or need them. Belief and shared collective desires *create* reality.

Support, caring and a healthy environment will take a national commitment and understanding that not only is this necessary today, but will positively influence and help the entire society given time. We need real leadership which has the intelligence to see that many elements of this society are working against the collective welfare and wholesomeness of society. Can we really justify spending $120 billion a year for war machinery when a significant number of our population is literally being struck down by a fantastic array of disease states that are the result of disturbed ideas and lifestyles created by fear, boredom, hatred, and resentment? We need to embrace what is good and right for the collective whole rather than laying blame. If we are to attain health and freedom, we must see this as an outgrowth of mental clarity where our actions and behavior patterns are our own and not impulses coming from a variety of hypnotic suggestions which continuously give the message "*more* is better." If we do not get control of our technology, it will "destroy" us, at least temporarily.

The healing community will operate within the laws of nature, trying to reestablish communion within oneself which will translate into communion with nature. As man becomes more conscious, he will intuitively understand his relationship with nature and his fellow man.

This may sound idealistic, however, not only are these concepts reasonable, but immediately necessary for healing to take place. The doctor of today not only has to work against his own higher nature in a competitive field of specialists, but must continuously be a scholar, scanning endless paper work, battling hostile and dissatisfied patients, working under conditions in and out of the hospital settings which do not allow him to enjoy and relax. The physician of today is as harried, as uptight and relatively as uncomfortable as those people he is trying to help. It really comes down to the nature of our work; better yet, how we individually and collectively use our energies. This comes down to choices which determine the course of our daily lives. Since we are inherently creative, even when we are doing nothing, we may appreciate that is simply a matter of redirecting our energies toward those endeavors which create satisfaction. And satisfaction is really communication. We are always the center of our own universe, supported by an infinite energy system. Call it life. Call it the self, call it God, call it the creative intelligence. Everything which exists is an aspect of this infinite, universal energy. It is the great machine behind all the action and yet it lives within all things. We are living in the middle of a phenomenal, mental universe, and it is our responsibility to create what is positive and beautiful; to enhance ourselves and thereby enhance others. This life is always working towards its own conscious evolution, and so are we. The breakthrough comes when we begin to be conscious of this evolution and realize that the cosmos is a "Dance of Life," supported by LOVE which has no beginning and no end. Perhaps it has created itself for its own enjoyment!!

Bibliography

Philosophy

Case, Paul Foster, *The Tarot: A Key to the Wisdom of the Ages.* Richmond, Virginia: Macoy Publishing Co., 1947.

Case, Paul Foster, *The Book of Tokens.* Los Angeles: Builders of the Adytum, 1960.

Chidhavananda, Swami, *The Bhagavad Gita* Tamil Nadu, India: Sri Ramakrisna Tapouanam, 1965.

Holy Scriptures. Philadelphia: The Jewish Publication Society of America, 1917.

Neville, *Your Faith Is Your Fortune.* Santa Monica, CA: DeVorss & Co., 1941.

Jung, C. G., *Psychology and Alchemy: Collected Works*, vol. 12, 2nd ed. Princeton, N.J.: Princeton University Press, 1944.

Bailey, Alice A., *Esoteric Healing.* New York. Lucis Publishing Co., 1953.

Rawson, Philip, and Laszlo Legeza, *Tao: The Eastern Philosophy of Time and Change.* New York: Avon Books, 1973.

Rawson, Philip, *Tantra: The Indian Cult of Ecstasy.* New York: Avon Books, 1973.

Roberts, Jane, *Seth Speaks.* Englewood Cliffs, N.J.: Prentice-Hall, 1972.

Roberts, Jane, *The Nature of Personal Reality.* Englewood Cliffs, N.J.: Prentice-Hall, 1974.

Burke, Richard, *Cosmic Consciousness: A Study in the Evolution of the Human Mind.* Secaucus, N.J.: Citadel Press, 1973.

Lilly, John C., *The Center of the Cyclone.* New York: Bantam Books, 1972.

Keyes, Ken, Jr., *Handbook to Higher Consciousness.* Berkeley, CA: Living Love Center, 1973.

Graham, E. L., ed., *The Rainbow Book.* Berkeley, CA: Shambhala, 1975.

Williams, Paul, *Das Energi.* New York: Elektra Books, 1973.

Watts, Alan, *Cloud Hidden, Whereabouts Unknown.* New York: Pantheon, 1968.

Oyle, Irving, *The Healing Mind.* Millbrae, CA: Celestial Arts, 1975.

De Ropp, Robert S., *The Master Game.* New York: Dell, 1968.

Human Sexuality

Case, Paul Foster, *The Tarot: A Key to the Wisdom of the Ages.* Richmond, Virginia: Macoy Publishing Co., 1947.

Reich, Wilhelm, *The Function of the Orgasm.* New York: Farrar, Straus & Giroux, 1973.

Comfort, Alex, *The Joy of Sex.* New York: Simon and Schuster, 1972.

Nutrition

Li Shin-chen, F. Porter Smith, and G. A. Stuart, *Chinese Medicinal Herbs.* San Francisco: Georgetown Press, 1973.

Airola, Paavoo, *Are You Confused?* Phoenix, Arizona: Health Plus, 1971.

Lust, John B., *The Herb Book.* New York: Bantam, 1974.

Jesus, *The Essene Gospel of Peace.*

Kloss, Jethro, *Back to Eden.* Santa Barbara, CA: Woodbridge Press, 1972.

Case, Paul Foster, *The Tarot: A Key to the Wisdom of the Ages.* Richmond, Virginia: Macoy Publishing Co., 1947.

Rose, Jeanne, *Herbs and Things.* New York: Grosset & Dunlap, 1972.

Cancer

Bailey, Alice, *Esoteric Healing.* New York: Lucis Publishing Co., 1953.

Reich, Wilhelm, *The Cancer Biopathy.* New York: Noonday Press, 1948.

Oyle Irving, *The Healing Mind.* Millbrae, CA: Celestial Arts, 1974.

Case, Paul Foster, *The Tarot: A Key to the Wisdom of the Ages.* Richmond, Virginia: Macoy Publishing Co., 1947.

Roberts, Jane, *Seth Speaks.* Englewood Cliffs, N.J.: Prentice-Hall, 1972.

The Drug Society

De Ropp, Robert S., *Drugs and the Mind.* New York: Grove Press, 1957.

Lingeman, Richard R., *Drugs from A to Z*, 2nd rev. ed. New York: McGraw-Hill, 1969.

Li Shin-Chen, F. Porter Smith and G. A. Stuart, *Chinese Medicinal Herbs*. San Francisco: Georgetown Press, 1973.

Physician's Desk Reference. Oradell, N.J.: Medical Economics Co., 1975.

Krupp, Marcus A., and Milton Chatton, *Medical Diagnosis and Treatment*. Los Altos, CA: Lange Medical Publications, 1974.

Davidson, Sir Stanley, and John Macleod, *The Principles and Practice of Medicine*. 10th ed. New York: Longman, 1972.

Death and Dying

Evans-Wentz, W. Y., *The Tibetan Book of the Dead*. New York: Oxford University Press, 1960.

Huxley, Laura, *This Timeless Moment*. Millbrae CA: Celestial Arts, 1968.

Anxiety and Depression

Laing, R. D., *The Politics of Experience*. New York: Pantheon, 1967.

Lilly, John C., *The Center of the Cyclone*. New York: Bantam, 1973.

Jung, C. G., *Freud and Psychoanalysis*. Princeton, N.J.: Princeton University Press, 1961.

Henderson, David, and R. D. Gillespie, *Textbook of Psychiatry for Students and Practitioners*, 10th ed. New York: Oxford University Press, 1969.

Netter, Frank, M.D., *The Nervous System*. Summit, New Jersey: The CIBA Collection of Medical Illustrations, 1972.

Netter, Frank, M.D., *The Endocrine System.* Summit, New Jersey: The CIBA Collection of Medical Illustrations, 1972.

Hospitals Today, Healing Centers Tomorrow

Bonny, Helen L., and Louis Savary, *Music and Your Mind: Listening with a new Consciousness.* New York: Harper & Row, 1973.

Case, Paul Foster, *The Tarot: A Key to the Wisdom of the Ages.* Richmond, Virginia: Macoy Publishing Co., 1947.

Graham, E. L., ed., *The Rainbow Book.* Berkeley, CA: Shambhala, 1975.

Kloss, Jethro, *Back to Eden.* Santa Barbara, CA: Woodbridge Press, 1972.

Suzuki, Shunryu, ed. by Trudy Dixon, *Zen Mind, Beginner's Mind.* New York: John Weatherhill, 1970.

Music

Halpern, Steve, *Spectrum Suite.* Palo Alto, CA: Spectrum Research Institute.

Inter-Dimensional Music, *IASOS.* Corte Madera, CA: Unity Records, 1975.

Wholistic Healing Center

The San Francisco Medical Research Foundation is a scientific nonprofit organization dedicated to using various time-tested techniques to prevent and cure various dis-ease manifestations which are psychosomatic in nature. It will be implicit within this organization that we (the staff) will assist in the process of healing, recognizing that we can and do determine our state of health by our attitudes and daily living habits. This center will work as a mutual cooperative foundation which will work both through didactic teaching and experiential techniques. We will treat the person wholistically, working on both the psyche and the soma, recognizing the immediate and direct relationship between the two.

This foundation also recognizes the profound effect environment has upon behavior and feeling and will apply the use of color and sound in a scientific manner to help induce states of profound relaxation whereby the patient will experience the deeper currents and feelings of his/her being. Direct feedback through the monitoring of the EKG, respiration, pulse and EEG will indicate the various effects upon the physiology of the body. There will also be indepth questioning to determine how the person views his experience and life subjectively, and we will quantiate both the subjective and objective data within a scientific framework to give a true picture of what health means to the individual.

The fundamental concepts and ideas of this center have been worked out in *Medicine Today, Healing Tomorrow*, and the book will serve as the basis for the treatment center.

I am currently president of the newly formed San Francisco Medical Research Foundation. As a non-profit organization, we are dependent upon donations and grants from private, corporate, and government sources. We are also open to establishing contact with other organizations or institutions involved in wholistic healing; we feel that communication and the sharing of ideas and knowledge are an intimate part of the growth process.

San Francisco Medical Research Foundation, Inc.
P. O. Box 7583
Rincon Annex
San Francisco, CA 94120
(415) 397-5753

BOOKS OF RELATED INTEREST

THE HEALING MIND, controversial, disturbing, fascinating first book by noted lecturer and medical researcher Dr. Irving Oyle, describes what is known about the mysterious ability of the mind to heal the body. 128 pages, soft cover, $4.95

SELECTIVE AWARENESS by Dr. Peter H.C. Mutke demonstrates the power of selective awareness in reprogramming negative thought/emotion patterns to promote physical health, healing, and the undoing of destructive habits such as overeating, smoking, insomnia, and pain. 240 pages, soft cover, $4.95

THE PAIN GAME by internationally known neurosurgeon C. Norman Shealy teaches the reader to break the chronic pain habit through the technique of balancing the body's physiology to achieve emotional attunement. 156 pages, soft cover, $4.95

TIME, SPACE AND THE MIND by Dr. Irving Oyle explores the mind's incredible ability to switch off time/space as the single most powerful healing tool available to humanity. 128 pages, soft cover, $4.95

In THE HEALING ENVIRONMENT Cristina Ismael presents a real alternative to traditional and institutionalized medicine: "By healing ourselves with and through the environment, we begin the process of healing the environment itself." 156 pages, soft cover, $4.95

In MAGIC, MYSTICISM AND MODERN MEDICINE, Dr. Irving Oyle paints engrossing staccato scenarios of his experiences as Director of an experimental health service doing research in holistic healing. 128 pages soft cover, $3.95

THE COMPLETE BOOK OF ACUPUNCTURE by Dr. Stephen Thomas Chang provides basic philosophy and practical applications of acupuncture for both laymen and physicians. Introduction by Dolph B. Ornstein. 252 pages, soft cover, $6.95

Stanley Krippner and Alberto Villoldo's REALMS OF HEALING presents a scientific exploration of non-medical healing and healers around the world, with emphasis on current laboratory research in the USA, the USSR, Brazil and Canada. 252 pages, soft cover, $6.95

Available at your local book or department store or directly from the publisher. To order by mail, send check or money order to:

Celestial Arts
231 Adrian Road
Suite MPB
Millbrae, California 94030

Please include 50 cents for postage and handling. California residents add 6% tax.